SENSORY EVALUATION OF APPEARANCE OF MATERIALS

A symposium
sponsored by ASTM
Committee E-12 on Appearance of
Materials, and Committee E-18 on
Sensory Evaluation of Materials
and Products
AMERICAN SOCIETY FOR
TESTING AND MATERIALS
Philadelphia, Pa., 24–25 Oct. 1972

ASTM SPECIAL TECHNICAL PUBLICATION 545
P. N. Martin and R. S. Hunter,
symposium co-chairmen

List price $19.75
04-545000-36

AMERICAN SOCIETY FOR TESTING AND MATERIALS
1916 Race Street, Philadelphia, Pa. 19103

Library of Congress Catalog Card Number: 73-87353

NOTE

The Society is not responsible, as a body,
for the statements and opinions
advanced in this publication.

Printed in Baltimore, Md.
December 1973

Foreword

Because of the overlapping interest of ASTM Committees E-12 on Appearance of Materials and E-18 on Sensory Evaluation of Materials and Products in vision and appearance, they have maintained liaison for many years, and joint sponsorship of this symposium was very appropriate. For Committee E-12 the symposium effort represented an extension beyond instrumental measurements, which had received most of their attention. For Committee E-18 it was a follow-up to ASTM Special Technical Publication 433, "Basic Principles of Sensory Evaluation" (1968), which included a chapter on vision and general chapters applying to all the senses. W. H. Danker, who was Chairman of Subcommittee E-18.02 during the early planning in 1970 and 1971, was largely responsible for the initial proposal for a joint effort of the two committees and the later proposal that this effort take the form of a symposium. W. J. Kiernan, who was Chairman of Committee E-12 in 1970, gave enthusiastic support to the proposed project and contributed many valuable suggestions for getting it underway.

The Chairmen of Committees E-12 and E-18 when the symposium was presented in 1972 were H. K. Hammond III and F. Sullivan. The Inter-Society Color Council also cooperated. P. N. Martin and R. S. Hunter presided as the symposium co-chairmen. Session chairmen included W. H. Danker, H. K. Hammond, R. S. Hunter, and O. R. Volk. Other members of the symposium task force were Mary W. Jenkins, J. W. Johnston, E. D. Kilmer, Angela C. Little, E. P. Rubacky, H. Stone, and R. M. Teates.

Related
ASTM Publications

Basic Principles of Sensory Evaluation, STP 433 (1968), $5.75 (04-433000-36)

Contents

Introduction

The field of sensory evaluation of materials is increasing in importance because of the present economic emphasis on consumer needs and wants. Foods are one line of products which obviously are rated critically on the sensory responses of human beings. There are many other materials which consumers use, however, in which human preferences and human responses are of major importance.

The papers in this publication deal with the human evaluation of the appearance characteristics of these various materials. It was planned and sponsored by ASTM Committees E-12 on Appearance of Materials and E-18 on Sensory Evaluation of Materials and Products. Committee E-12 is concerned primarily with direct physical measurement of properties, such as tristimulus color, which are related to human vision by established formulas. Committee E-18, on the other hand, works with statistical techniques for relating physically measured attributes to human responses by correlation and regression analyses.

One purpose of the symposium was to report the state of the art in psychophysical analyses of appearance; that is, methods of correlating physical measurements of light with sensory ratings of appearance. Another purpose was to provide a forum for describing recent developments and trends in these areas.

The symposium was planned to include the following topics: (1) mechanism of vision, (2) psychology of appearance of materials, (3) estimation of subjective impressions, (4) correlation of the objective facts with subjective impressions, and (5) anomalies, pitfalls, problems, and a look at the future. Speakers were invited and obtained from outside, as well as from within ASTM.

We believe that the papers presented in this publication will be of interest and value to anyone concerned with color or other aspects of appearance of foods, beverages, textile fabrics for clothing and furnishings, plastics, paint and other coatings, architectural materials, paper, and other products. Psychologists, educators, scientists, those in the advertising, marketing, market research fields, and others concerned with consumer responses should be interested.

This publication contains two state-of-art-papers. One gives a picture of the eye as the device for converting light to signals for analysis by the brain. The second is an up-to-date summary of what ASTM has accomplished in the development of consensus approved methods for measuring appearance attributes by instrument.

Two of the papers are concerned with appearance ratings of foodstuffs; one with visual preferences in textile materials; and several with the complex statistical techniques used to establish relationships between human judgments and physically measureable variables. Thus, two of the papers are concerned only with statistical methods, not with appearance. The question of how to assess important aspects of visual appearance is approached from a number of viewpoints in the papers.

R. S. Hunter
Hunter Associates Lab., Inc.,
Fairfax, Va.

P. N. Martin
Consumer Products Division,
SCM Corporation,
New York, N.Y.

J. W. Johnston, Jr.[1]

Mechanism of Vision—A Review

REFERENCE: Johnston, J. W., Jr., "**Mechanism of Vision–A Review,**" *Sensory Evaluation of Appearance of Materials, ASTM STP 545,* American Society for Testing and Materials, 1973, pp. 3-17.

ABSTRACT: The human retinal image is a pattern of light and dark that differs from a picture within the central nervous system. A remarkable characteristic is the "saccade," a very fast flicking of the eyeballs such that a new focus of the image is formed on the cone cells of the central pit every few milliseconds. The saccade is especially important to reading when the day-vision cones function. The night-vision rods do not add much to day vision but are a fourth mechanism in respect to the three kinds of cones which enable the brain to distinguish contrasts between spectral hues. Despite the infinite variety of textures and settings with which colors are often perceived, there is a limited degree of color constancy of objects under varying conditions of brightness, size, and shape.

KEY WORDS: senses, perception, visual perception, memory, surfaces, images

That part of the nervous system of man which serves the visual processes is more subtle than the notion as was implied by the old "image theory" started by Johannes Kepler. He wrote in 1604 A.D. that the human eye was like a camera. Now it is understood that the retinal image is a pattern of light and dark that differs from a picture within the nervous system. Whenever people speak of a "photographic memory" they are reflecting Kepler's analogy, but the truth is that perception and memory are an integrative process with spatial and temporal parameters that are unique attributes of the nervous system.

Although binocular vision yields a more accurate depth perception than one-eyed vision, they are fundamentally alike. The world looks much the same with one eye closed as it does with both of them open [*1*].[2] In order to appreciate the components of the modern theory of vision, we can think directly about the appearance of real objects and surfaces that are illuminated ordinarily by sunshine or lamplight. Inquiry into how these reflected patterns affect us has

[1] Associate professor of Physiology, retired, Georgetown University Medical School, Washington, D. C. 20007; now at 8940 Jones Mill Rd., Chevy Chase, Md. 20015.

[2] The italic numbers in brackets refer to the list of references appended to this paper.

been termed "ecological optics" and has revealed important facts about perception. It is an optics in which point sources, homogeneous fields, and the other basic elements of classical optics rarely appear. Instead, our visual world consists mostly of surfaces at various angles and in various relations to one another [*2*].

Anatomy

That the area of clear vision on the retina (Fig. 1) is severely limited to a stationary eye is important to an understanding of vision. This can only be grasped by noting the fovea. It is a small focal region of the retinal macula that contains a pure population of cones which is approximately 4 mm^2 [*3*]. It is a pit that is packed tightly with cones, one of the two kinds of visual receptors, that function in daylight (only) and also has the unique function of discriminating the various wavelengths that produce the sensation of color. At any moment only a small region around the fixation point will be clearly seen. Thus, most of a typed page will be seen by the peripheral receptors, which means that it is hazily visible at best (Fig. 1)! It is only in the fovea that the small, packed cones, appropriately organized by the nerve fibers over which impulses travel, yield a high degree of visual acuity (see the following). Because of the saccadic movements, one sees the page or scene as a whole without any apparent discontinuity in space or time (see the following). The visual world is somehow constructed of information taken in during many fixations.

The vertical midline section of the eyeball presents the salient anatomical characteristics. A ray of white light from a point source penetrates the outer cornea, a clear fluid, the pupil, and the biconcave lens. Other light rays, parallel to the optical axis, are focused by convergence so that, as they pass through the rather viscous medium that fills the eyeball, they produce a minute light spot on the retina at the fovea. During day vision, it is the cones in an area of less than 3 mm diameter which give rise to impulses; while in darkness, the stimulus-intensity is too weak to affect the cones and the slender rods become the sole functional receptors. Ultimately, the impulses (neural signals) are transmitted to the optic nerve and, thence, to a relay nucleus in the brainstem.

A complicated cytology within the retina, however, needs explanation because of the important bearing it has upon modern theory [*4*]. Note that the rods and cones end upon a thin pigmented membrane (Fig. 2), which is attached to the inner coat of the eyeball. Note how the path of the light rays is through the retina to its remote side which is away from the lens. Therefore, the electrical impulses move in the direction of the center of the eyeball, principally through two neurons, the second in line being the all-important ganglion cell. The cones in the fovea form a direct chain linkage with the ganglion cells while the cones and rods of the peripheral retina converge upon the bipolar neurons in ratios of 3:1 or 4:1. These peripheral bipolar cells connect with ganglion cells in

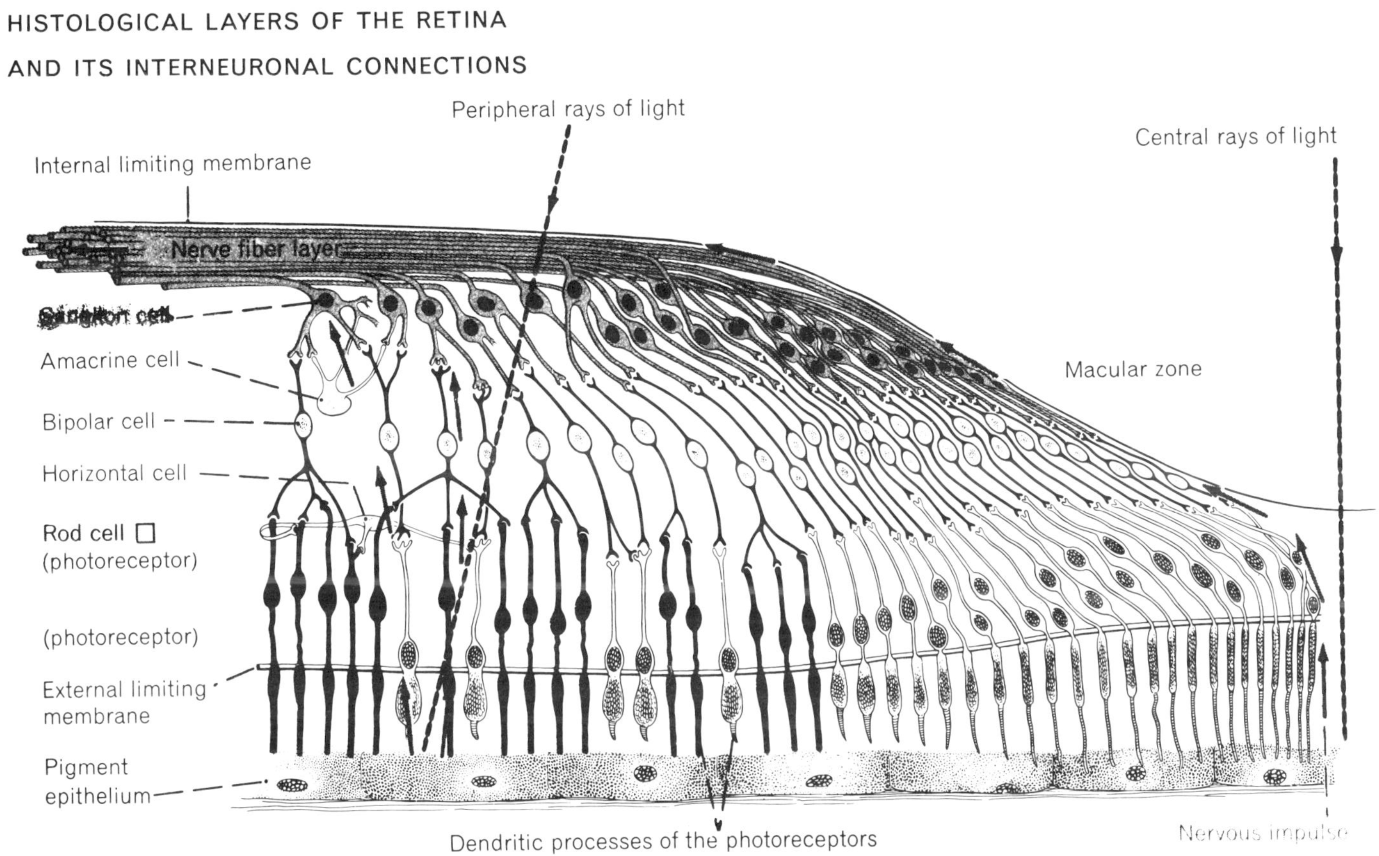

FIG. 1–*Microscopic diagram of the retina (by B. Melloni,* What's New, *No. 222, 1961; courtesy of Abbott Laboratories, Inc.*).

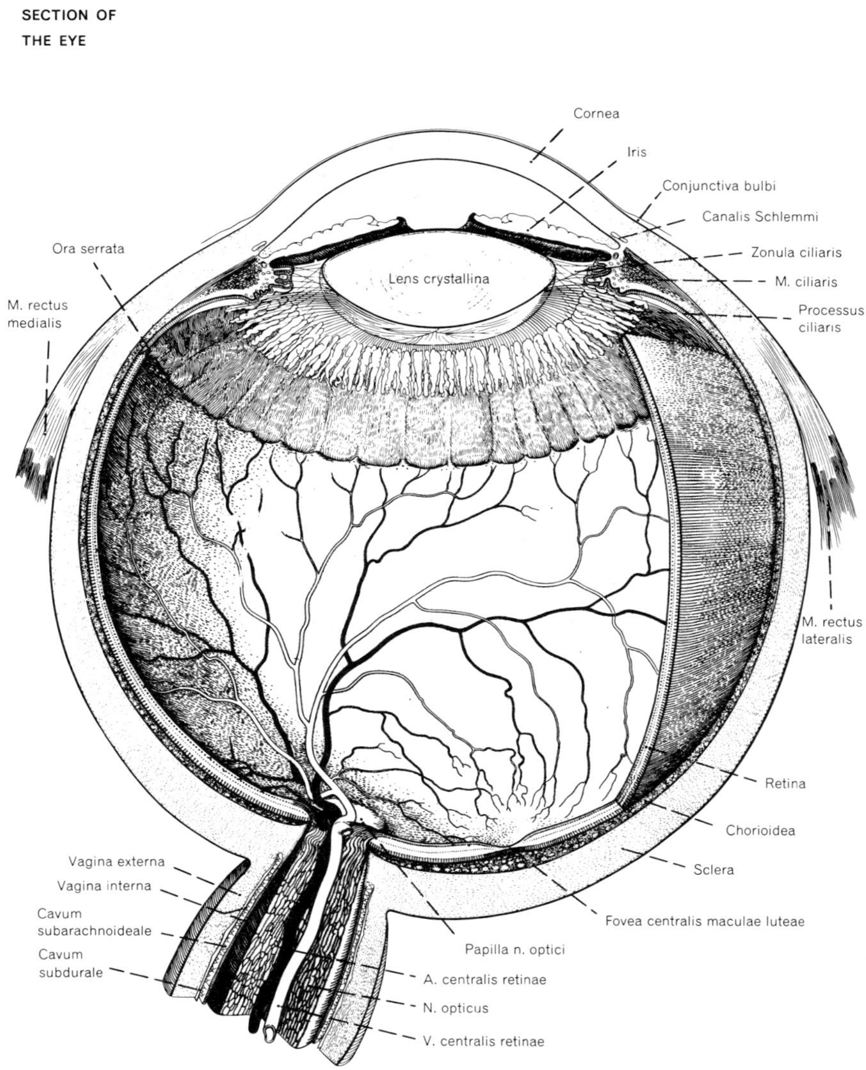

FIG. 2–*The layers of the eyeball and its optical axis; note the fovea in the retina–the optical focus or fixation point (by B. Melloni,* What's New, *No. 222, 1961; courtesy of Abbott Laboratories, Inc.*).

a variety of ways that enable a unit of either cones or rods to transmit the impulse to more than one ganglion cell. This elaborate transmission system is further influenced by feed-back neurons, the amacrines which transmit impulses between adjacent ganglion cells.

To summarize this complex functional aspect, the anatomical division between the central and peripheral retina rests upon the different accumulation of ganglion cells in the two regions. Ganglion cells are small and densely packed in six to seven rows at the edge of the cup-shaped foveal depression and reduce to one row at the outer margin of the area. However, ganglion cells in the periphery form a continuous, occasionally broken, single layer. Furthermore, the innervation density of the receptive surface (the number of receptors per unit area) means that each ganglion cell defines a retinal receptive unit; that is, the population of receptors distributed over an area of retinal surface which is connected to the brain by a single fiber [3]. In considering the brain parts serving vision, the ganglion cell may then be taken as the representative member of the peripheral surface.

Higher Brain Centers

Extensions of retinal ganglion neurons in the optic nerves make connections in a pair of relay stations in the brainstem, the lateral geniculate bodies. The optic nerves cross each other just under the brain and provide for some fibers of a given receptive unit to pass to the opposite hemisphere of the brain while the remainder pass to the hemisphere of the same side; that is, right eye to right hemisphere, for instance. The ganglion neurons connect at these bodies with the next neurons in the series which, in turn, make their upper connections with cerebral neurons situated on the inner rear surface of the cerebral mantel. The extensions of neurons in the lateral geniculate bodies transmit to cerebral neurons situated on each side of the calcarine fissure (an anatomical landmark), the so-called visual cortex.

Optical and Physiological Functions

One of the two great abilities of the eye when it is adapted to daylight viewing is the detection and discrimination of fine detail. The other ability is the perception of colors which will be described after the photochemistry of the visual pigments. Both of these functions are a property of the foveal cones which were just described.

In respect to the target direction and resolving power, the most important direction corresponds to the center of the fovea, for here the anatomical and functional organization of the retina is most favorable for good resolution. Normally, the two eyes will be positioned to image the object of regard in the centers of the foveas. Thus, the primary line of sight is from the object to the cones of the fovea. When a person with good vision holds a human hair before him at arms length, it is perfectly discernable as a cylindrical object and is a familiar choice of target for demonstrating resolving power.

The retinal image is not a point-by-point replica of the target no more than a perfect optical instrument forms a point image (Fig. 3)[5]. The light is spread coming from a point object into a diffraction pattern whose size is inversely related to the pupil aperture. We see best when the diameter of the pupil is 2 mm or less and poorly when the diameter is more than 5 mm. A point object such as a star will, even under the best conditions, spread its light over an appreciable retinal region. When two point sources such as two stars are close together, each will produce its own light spread, but the two light spots will summate: what a retinal receptor responds to is the sum of all the light reaching it from all sources and over its whole acceptance area. The graph-shape of the summed light distribution from two closely adjacent point sources differs insignificantly from that of a single, brighter target, and it is therefore impossible to make the distinction between a single and a double light source. If the two point sources are now separated, a graph of the intensity spots on the retina will show two distinct humps with a trough between them. The condition for resolution has now been reached provided, however, that the receptor mosaic (unit) has a "grain" such that the darker band between two brighter spots causes them to fall on individual mosaic units, and that the physiological pathway from each of these units is capable of transmitting independent signals (impulses). This example illustrates the factors involved in the resolution of spatial details or visual acuity: optical (point-spread function), anatomical (receptor units), and functional (independent pathways for transmitting signals). It has been accepted

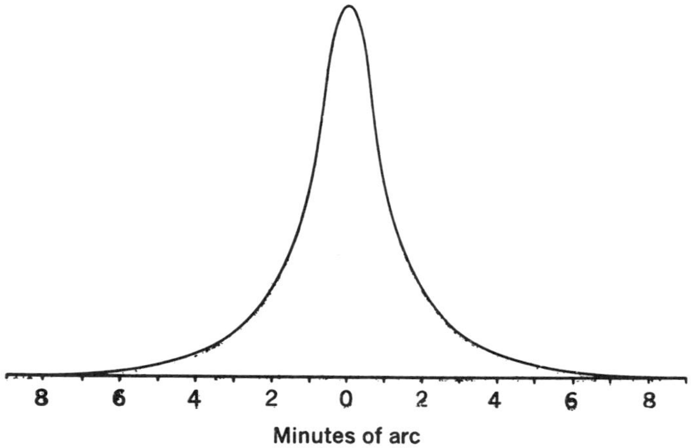

FIG. 3–*Light spread in human eye. Even in best state of focus, the optics of eye spreads the light from a line source over a finite distance of fovea*[2].

for at least a century that normal visual acuity is 1 min of arc [3]; that is separation of two stars by 1 min of arc leads to the sensation of two stars, and by less than 1 min of arc to a sensation of one star as diagrammed in Fig. 3.

Day and Night Vision

An understanding of functional microscopic anatomy has been obtained from electrophysiological experiments in which a minute pick-up electrode is placed either against the surface of the neuron or inside of its cell body. As the stimulus puts an adequate amount of energy into the receptor, a photochemical reaction occurs that gives rise to the impulse under certain conditions. The rods contain the chemical rhodopsin which interacts with all visible wavelengths; their reactions vary only in amplitude as the stimulus-intensity varies [4]. In very weak illumination, the cones do not respond and one "sees" with the peripheral retina. Convergent neural pathways of rods to ganglion cells yield summation of the impulses which this layer of the retina can process. When the eye is adapted to darkness, the functional pathways of the impulses serve to detect the objects. When one receives the usual amount of reflected illumination of daylight or indoor lighting, the functional pathways change to the light-adapted state which has a theoretical advantage for the detection of a border in the retinal stimulus.

It may be that detection of a border requires different discharge rates for ganglion cells that are close together but on opposite sides of the border. A little-understood feature of the nervous system is the way certain neurons will respond positively to the impulse while others respond negatively, a mutual inhibition between the central and peripheral parts of the receptive field. This seems to enhance this difference between discharge rates of ganglion cells on opposite sides of the border, thus improving the ability of the retina to detect borders by daylight. This flexibility of the functional pathways through the retina seems to change to meet the demands of different conditions.

Visual Pigments

In order to appreciate the receptors, it is necessary to consider the photochemistry of the visual pigments concentrated within the outer segments of the rods and cones. In some way it is these processes that are involved with the origins of the neural electrical impulses (signals) that the brain integrates into shadings of light and dark, forms and colors. Two photo-pigments have been isolated and identified, the rhodopsin of the rods and the iodopsin of certain cones, while at least the existence of two additional cone pigments has been demonstrated by spectrophotometry.

Rhodopsin and iodopsin molecules are a combination of a protein (generically termed opsins) and a chromophore (retinene$_1$) like other pigments. Retinene$_1$ is common to both molecules and is borne by an opsin, so it is the protein component which is different for each visual pigment [6].

Inasmuch as it has been easier to extract rhodopsin for isolated investigation, most detailed information has been gleaned about the rods (which primarily subserve the dark-adapted eye). Rhodopsin has been extracted from the retinas of several vertebrate species, whereas iodopsin has been only extracted with difficulty from the pure cone retinas of chickens. Consequently, the very rapid changes of form of rhodopsin after the light stimulus has impinged upon the molecule serve as the basis of a brief, leading explanation. Activation first causes the chromatophore $retinene_1$ to be isomerized and then the protein opsin changes form. This is followed in man by a true bleaching reaction in which the molecule splits into its two component parts. Then the $retinene_1$ is reduced to Vitamin A_1 by the enzyme alcohol dehydrogenase working with the coenzyme diphosphopyridinenucleotide, and finally much of Vitamin A_1 migrates out of the outer segments of the rods into the pigment epithelium for storage. This epithelium is one cell thick and lies between the receptor layer and the inner surface of the eyeball.

In this way, more and more rhodopsin is broken down in the presence of light stimulation and is finally resynthesized to $retinene_1$ by conversion in the dark from retinene to the original form by an enzyme. As these chemical reactions give off energy, the final step is a spontaneous recombination of $retinene_1$ and opsin within the outer segment.

Iodopsin's breakdown and resynthesis has the same major reactions, but details of the intermediate steps are not known. Spectrophotometry of the living human cones suggests that iodopsin corresponds with a pigment that is sensitive to the red wavelengths[*4*]. This technique also demonstrates the existence of pigments that are sensitive to green and blue wavelengths. Inasmuch as only a few human cones have been studied, we must not expect too much of the biochemical evidence, but it does agree with similar studies of the rhesus monkey and goldfish. In the latter species ample sized samples of the three groups of cones have established this primary receptive mechanism. A central problem awaiting further spectrophotometric measurements is whether each type of cone contains a single visual pigment, or whether some cones contain mixtures. Cones have been measured which contained mainly red-sensitive pigment mixed with a minor amount of green-sensitive pigment. This merely points up the possibility that some of the cones, especially red-sensitive ones, do contain mixtures of visual pigments[7].

The trapping of an adequate amount of light energy, the quantum, by a molecule of pigment leads also to the sequential excitation of the receptor which is the principal functional event of perception in the retina. Perhaps the steps are a direct photoelectric transduction that releases electrons or other charges carried from the photopigment molecule. Many electrophysiological experiments have revealed several electrical "waves," one of which may be the receptor potential. Never-the-less, this idea of the "triggering mechanism" has not been proved. Therefore, one needs to consider the alternate possibility that one of the events in the breakdown of the pigment "triggers" the electrical activity. This notion implies a double transduction: photochemical and chemoelectrical!

In respect to a quantum of the stimulus, a human rod can be excited by the absorption of a single quantum, but this does not result in a threshold sensation. At least two rods and perhaps as many as eight have to be excited during the period of time within which temporal summation can occur in order for a human being to sense light [*3*].

Color Vision

Turning now to the three-primaries color vision theory, it is necessary to introduce psychological considerations from the start. This is due to recent findings about color coding in man as well as the house cat [*7*]. In respect to the first trichromatic theory which supposed three distinct primaries, and the just-mentioned photopigments within the cones (like iodopsin), a distinction must be drawn between the theory as a true one involving assumptions about visual mechanisms, and a "trichromatic theory" as an empirical generalization about color matching. The latter idea may be laid down in a weaker, qualitative form valid over a very wide range of conditions of observation, or in a stronger, quantitative form of narrower application. The concept of a one-to-one serial anatomical relationship of the foveal cones and the neural pathways to the brain cortex at the back of the head was deemed insufficient to explain color vision. The question arose as to whether a given foveal cone was responsive to a given wavelength of light in one state of activity and a simple light-or-dark response (achromatic) in another. This idea does not, however, support the outmoded Duplicity Color Vision Theory [*6*], as there seems to be a difference, for example, of yellow-blue and red-green versus white-black processes. This thinking portends that the tools of electrophysiology may be supplemented by those of cellular chemistry. When this newer methodology is developed the pigments could be discretely investigated in place; for example, within the receptors.

Deductive Logic and the Overview

Another point of the evidence for color vision is the considerable overlap between the difference spectra of the three receptor classes. Thus, a wavelength of light will stimulate at least two and in some cases three of the cone classes. This means that at the receptor level there is a response code for color since each wavelength of light will elicit a unique ratio of responses among the three fundamental receptor classes. Hence, electrophysiologists have placed single fiber electrodes in such numbers in an animal preparation that a battery of impulses can be simultaneously transmitted to a computer so that a variety of discharge patterns caused by controlled light stimuli may be viewed as the decisive indicators of chemical coding.

There is weak evidence of at least one pair of opponent colors, the "mass action" theory. First data provided the direct evidence of three kinds of cones that are reasonably consistent in their properties with the hypothetical components of early or 19th century trichromatic theory. Direct measurements were made with a microspectrophotometer of single parafoveal cones of man that yielded difference spectra of the visual pigments which revealed the presence of (at least) three groups of cones, red, green, and blue-sensitive. Few cones have yet been measured, however, in this way to define the reliability of absorption maxima. Stiles may have found evidence for the red mechanism of man to involve the operation of both the red and green-sensitive pigments by means of mass action spectra and they now have the force of absorption spectra of the color vision pigments [*4*]; their maxima lie at about 430, 540, and 575 millimicrons. It is interesting to note, therefore, that the rods constitute a fourth independent mechanism in the range of intensities in which both rods and cones are active. Neutral gray sensations are stimulated by rods with the result that rod vision does no more than to desaturate the colors we see without apparently altering their hues.

Perception of Size

Perception of size (Fig. 4) relies heavily on cues provided by a textured surface. The five disks in the illustration, if seen alone, would appear to lie in one plane and be of different sizes. Against the apparently receding surface, however, they seem to lie in five different planes. Since each disk masks the same amount of surface texture, there is a tendency to see them as being equal in size ([*1*] figure after J. J. Gibson of Cornell University).

It is a fact that the sizes of real objects are almost always perceived accurately in spite of the linear dependence of retinal-image size on distance "size constancy." Since one does not see one's own retina, the apparent size of an object is determined by information from the entire incoming light pattern, particularly by certain properties of the input that remain constant with change of the object's location [*8*].

One may appreciate that our visual field has a microstructure because most target surfaces have some kind of texture. The light thus reflected carries vital information about the layout of environmental objects. When a microstructure of a surface slants away from the observer, it is represented on the retina as a gradient of density. In accordance with principles of perspective, the gradient carries information about the orientation of the surface.

This example may be misleading simply because it assumes a stationary condition of the eyes, whereas this is by no means a characteristic of human vision. Normal eyes are rarely still for long as they commonly flick from one

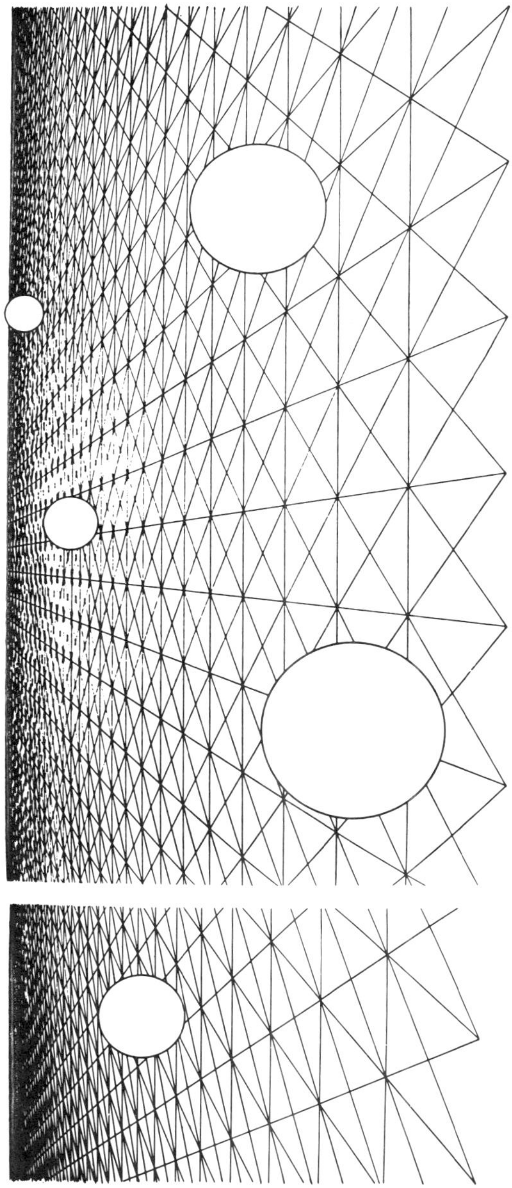

FIG. 4–*Perception of size relies heavily upon cues provided by a textured surface* [1].

position to another, an attribute called a "saccade"[1]. Saccades usually take less than a twentieth of a second, but they happen several times each second in reading and may be just as frequent when a picture or an actual scene is being inspected. This means that there is a new retinal image every few hundred milliseconds.

A current theory of vision holds that one sees a composite based on information accumulated over a period of time. Information from past fixations is used together with information from the present fixation to determine what is seen. But if perception is a temporarily extended act, some storage of information, some kind of memory, must be involved in it!

Brain Function

The neural pathways of the visual impulses are relevant to the relatively complex ability to discriminate patterns primarily at more central levels of the visual system; namely, in the brainstem and cerebral cortex. This ability requires some type of learning process that must be started early in life[1]. Hence, one should appreciate that sensory physiology is different from all other fields of physiology in that its problems are closely related to, or even identical with, certain problems of psychology, epistemology, and logic. One might state that sensory physiology and psychology are virtually indistinguishable. By characterizing the lateral geniculate bodies as "relay stations" it is probable that they affect the incoming signals as the first stage of integration and analysis. The terminations of optic fibers with the next neurons-in-line is sharply circumscribed according to the receptive retinal units.

Just how the retinal units are related to the visual cerebral cortex is not clear, but it may reasonably be assumed that it furnishes an orderly central replication of the two-dimensional resolving power of the retina. It is certain that each single incoming fiber connects with more than one fiber. Just what happens next is complicated, especially in the cortex, by the anatomical connections between neurons through a wide-spread branching or via smaller neurons that form connections between fiber pathways. Thus, it is possible that the signals are distributed over a population of neurons much larger than the original receiving population and the farther neurons bring about a functional multiplication and overlap whose extent and character would also depend on the intrinsic function of the connections; namely, on their excitatory or inhibitory nature.

The further integration and analysis of the coded signals by the cerebral mantel would next occur in neurons of the primary visual cortex. There has occurred a greater degree of convergence of impulses here and even more occurs beyond it in what are designated Visual Areas II and III. These intracortical transformations increase the functional specificity of these neurons towards the spatial configuration of the light stimulus falling on the retina and most likely towards other parameters of the stimulus as well.

An important idea about how the human brain determines discrimination of color is by the perception of differences among the responses of the three kinds of cones. What is implied is the perception of differences rather than the sheer perceptions of color stimuli. In passing, it is interesting to note that measurements of color discrimination indicate in general that visual discrimination of colors is, under the most favorable conditions, better than the best available physical detector.

Color Constancy

In real life our visual environment, like that of monkeys, is structured in terms of "objects" with fixed properties, such as size, brightness, color, shape, and position. It is appreciated that each object has a so-called color which is its capacity to modify the color of the light incident upon it. This is the basis of the "color constancy" principle. Under everyday conditions certain complex psychological factors that affect most object-color perceptions are largely independent of changes in illumination and viewing conditions. This is what is meant by the expression "color constancy." We find that responses to color are not affected by marked changes in brightness, size, shape, position, and distance. Furthermore, color (as well as size, brightness, shape, and many other properties of objects) is not markedly influenced by changes in illumination or in the character of the illuminant [*9*].

The monkey's lateral geniculate bodies' connections, and presumably man's, with the primary visual cerebral cortex guarantee an approximate constancy of the objects and their interrelations in the visual environment and provide the normal monkey with a visual world that has a remarkable degree of stability. Color constancy phenomena are largely confined to the surface and volume modes of color perception which are further classified as the illuminant, illumination, and film modes. These categories are quite arbitrary because of the infinite variety of textures and settings with which colors are often perceived [*8*].

Some modes of appearance can be recognized in a picture of a scene (which we may have experienced naturally). The steps of appearance which approach more and more an original scene are generally: picture or prints, transparency, stereo, motion pictures, sound motion picture, stereo-sound motion picture, and finally the original scene itself. Not expecting a change in the object, the observer is less likely to recognize changes in what he regards as part of the object—its color. Probably the most volatile and potent interpretive factor is the attitude of the observer. Attitude (and more generally, interest) comprises the internal control of attention, and by determining what is looked at and what is looked for, has much to do with what is actually seen or perceived.

A very practical fact concerns observers, or color judges, who have been specially instructed (in the "scaling" of color constancy) to have a normal, object-directed attitude. It is rare that a high degree of constancy occurs so that a rather limited degree is usual. Thus, the concept is weakly supported in practice probably because an analytical attitude disfavors color constancy. (Monkeys respond "intuitively" in controlled experiments.) Because of the limited constancy typical of attempts at measurement, expressions like partial color constancy, or regression toward the real object, are more accurately indicative of the observed facts than the usual unmodified expression, color constancy.

Since it is no longer possible to discuss color vision in the older, traditionally mechanistic manner because of the close affinity of sensory physiology and psychology, an idea is drawn from the Science of Hedonics (the study of likes and dislikes). Man's subjective responses do not conform to the principles of psychophysics as if they were various intensities of red and blue. In the real world an orangy color added to commercial orange juice lends a positive hedonic response. If the juice were colored a metallic blue, for example, many people would reject the product. Likewise, the skins of frankfurters are colored "appropriately" in order to impart an appetizing appearance. One could imagine how a premeditated "inappropriate" coloring of a product, printed illustration, or animated diagram could elicit a negative hedonic response. This notion implies counter propaganda that might serve a socially constructive end! In a subsequent chapter of this publication there is a treatment of "Appearance: Likes and Dislikes." This somewhat neglected science is carefully explained.

Conclusions

Inasmuch as this article is a review of salient literature on the anatomy, physiology, and psychology of vision, it is a set of conclusions. However, the reader should realize that the modern trichromatic theory has not yet achieved final acceptance for the human eye, as it has for the goldfish. Furthermore, the contributions of psychology force us to appreciate there are subtlies of brain function that have not been measured by the direct technique of electrophysiology. It is these properties of human vision that are passed over in some discussions of this subject.

References

[*1*] Neisser, Ulric, *Scientific American,* Vol. 219, 1968, pp. 204-214.

[*2*] Beck, Jacob, *Surface Color Perception,* Cornell University Press, Ithaca, N. Y., 1972.

[*3*] Mountcastle, V., *Medical Physiology,* Vol. II, C. V. Mosby Co., St. Louis, Mo., 1968.

[*4*] Wald, G. and Brown, P. K., "Sensory Receptors," Cold Spring Harbor Symposium on Quantitative Biology, Vol. 30.

[*5*] Westheimer, G., *Journal of the Optical Society of America,* Vol. 53, 1963, p. 90.

[*6*] de Reuck, A. V. S. and Knight, J., *Colour Vision, Physiology and Experimental Psychology,* Little, Brown & Co., Boston, 1965.

[7] Hurvich, L. M. and Jameson, D., "Color Vision and Color Coding," Chapter 2, *Perception and Its Disorders,* Vol. XLVIII, Research Publication A.R.N.M.D., 1970. pp. 12-25.

[8] *The Science of Color,* Committee on Colorimetry, Optical Society of America, New York, 1953.

[9] Burham, R. W., Hanes, R. M., and Bartleson, C. J., *Color, A Guide to Basic Facts and Concepts,* Wiley, New York, 1963.

R. S. Hunter [1]

Visually Perceived Attributes of the Appearance of Materials and ASTM Progress Toward Their Measurement

REFERENCE: Hunter, R. S., "**Visually Perceived Attributes of the Appearance of Materials and ASTM Progress Toward Their Measurement,**" *Sensory Evaluation of Appearance of Materials, ASTM STP 545,* American Society for Testing and Materials, 1973, pp. 18-34.

ABSTRACT: To analyze appearance attributes optically, one first separates the chromatic attributes from the geometric ones. The chromatic, or color, attributes may be represented in a variety of forms which start with the purely physical spectrophotometric curves. By incorporating the sensory processes of the human observer, one converts spectrophotometric data to colorimetric specification by use of the CIE Standard Observer and Coordinate System. To obtain analyses which relate closely to the observer's sensory impressions, one can convert CIE specifications to one of several opponent-colors (L,a,b-type) analyses or to hue, value, and chroma of the Munsell-type analyses. These sensory-related color specification systems can be used to locate points representing colors in three-dimensional coordinate systems. Geometric attributes are those related to the geometric manners in which objects and materials distribute light and are known by terms such as gloss, turbidity, texture, and the like. Measurement methods for many of the various geometric attributes have been developed.

Total instrumental analyses of the physical correlates of appearance are so complex that measurement is not feasible and is never attempted. There do exist, however, a large number of practical, useful methods for instrumentally measuring specific attributes of the appearance of materials. Many of these have been standardized in print by the American Society for Testing and Materials (ASTM), which now has the largest published collection of appearance analyses in existence. Although ASTM has accomplished much in promoting measurements of appearance attributes, there exist important requirements for test procedures not yet prepared. The technical state of the art has recently progressed so that ASTM should now be able to meet these unsatisfied requirements.

KEY WORDS: senses, perception, visual perception, glossimetry, colorimetry, chromaticity, appearance of materials

Visual recognition of objects is a major element of every sighted person's daily experience. Normally, the observer does not analyze the appearance of an

[1] President, Hunter Associates Laboratory, Inc., Fairfax, Va. 22030

object in terms of its optical properties, but relies on his previous experience, expectations, and specific concerns of the moment in evaluating appearance of what he sees as a totality. For example, the appearance of a steak in a super market is normally interpreted by the viewer in terms of characteristics which he has learned to associate with quality. Not until appearance measurement or control is needed does one become concerned with the optical nature of the attributes of appearance of materials.

The Measurable Attributes of Object Appearance

Chromatic and Geometric Attributes

Objects and materials are seen by how they affect the light that falls on them. The measurable attributes of appearance divide broadly into two categories: chromatic (having to do with color) and geometric (having to do with geometric distribution of light, gloss, haze, etc.). The chromatic or color attributes are by far the most important commercially, but it is necessary, when considering overall appearance and when selecting conditions for the measurement of color, that geometric characteristics of light distribution by the objects be considered.

Distinction Between Physical and Psychophysical Measurements of Appearance

A second important distinction in classifying appearance measurements is that between measurements of complete spectral and geometric distributions, which can be called physical, and those measurements of quantities chosen specifically to correlate with visual estimates. These latter are called psychophysical since they are physical measurements designed specifically to correlate with the various attributes of object appearance.

Table 1 is designed to summarize the distinctions between the physical and the psychophysical attributes of appearance as well as those between the chromatic and geometric. At the top in Table 1 are spectrophotometric curves giving physical analyses of the distribution of light responsible for color. In a second column are goniophotometric curves giving physical analyses of geometric distributions responsible for the geometric attributes such as gloss. In the next line below are the psychological or visual attributes of appearance which one normally sees and speaks of in his visual recognition of the corresponding attributes.

The third line in the table identifies the bases by which appearance correlating measurements are derived from the purely physical. Then in the bottom line are named the psychophysical quantities with symbols which are measured to give numbers correlating with the attributes seen visually.

Geometric Classes of Objects

To select geometric conditions for appearance measurement, objects and materials are divided into four classes depending on whether they only reflect

TABLE 1–*Distinctions between major color and geometric attributes in the appearance of objects.*

Category	Color Attributes	Geometric Attributes
Physical	Spectrophotometric curves 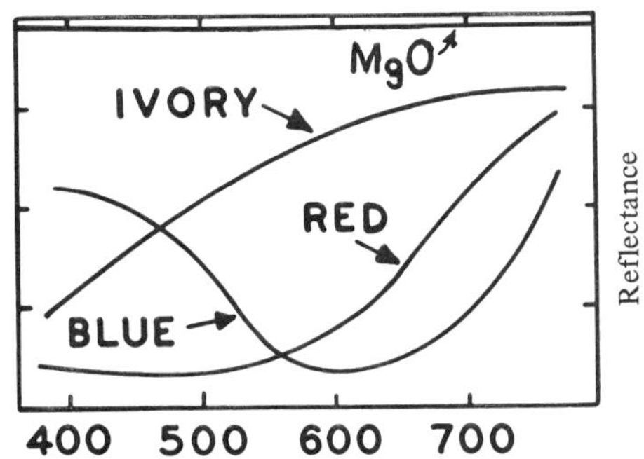 Wavelength, nm	Goniophotometric curves 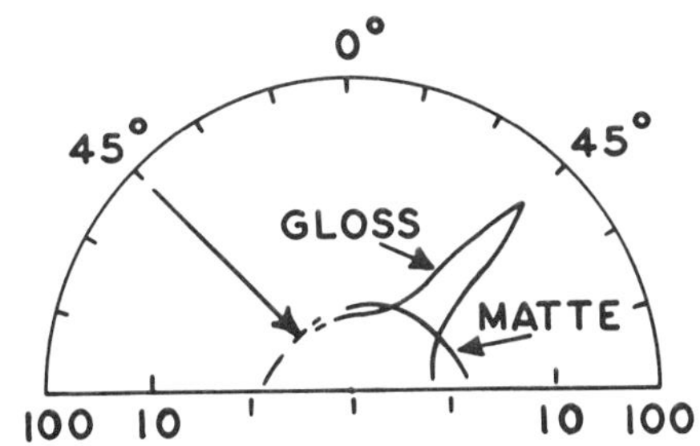 Reflection Factor
Psychological, (visual)	Color: Hue } chromaticity Saturation } Lightness or one of the geometric attributes in the next column	Luminous intensity: Lightness (by diffuse reflection) Shininess (by specular reflection) Lightness (by diffuse transmission) Transparency (by specular transmission)
Basis of psychophysical measurement	Ability of human observer to match color of any object by adding proper amount of three colored primary lights	Comparisons with ideal objects that either diffuse light perfectly or have perfect specular projection
Psychophysical quantities with symbols	Chromaticity (hue and saturation together) may be any of the following pairs of attributes: 1. chromaticity coordinates (x, y) 2. dominant wavelength (Λ) purity (p) 3. redness-greenness (a) yellowness-blueness (b)	Directional reflectance factor (R_d), or Lightness ($L = 10\sqrt{R_d}$) Gloss (R_s, G_s, G_c, G_i, etc.) Directional transmittance factor (T_d) Specular transmittance factor (T_s)

light or transmit light, and depending on whether they distribute most of the light that leaves them diffusely or specularly:

1. diffusely reflecting opaque non-metal surface,
2. specularly reflecting metallic surfaces,
3. translucent (diffusely transmitting) sheets, and
4. transparent films, sheets, and volumes.

Table 2 lists the four optical classes which result when one makes these separations and identifies the dominant geometric mode of light distribution and corresponding appearance attributes of each. The majority of products measured instrumentally are diffusely-reflecting non-metals. Thus, in Table 3, the ASTM methods of test specifically applicable to diffusely reflecting materials such as paint, plastic, and paper are separated from the methods used for other materials in Table 4.

Specific Attributes of Appearance

In Tables 3 and 4 which list the attributes of appearance and the ASTM methods of test for each, it is seen that there exists a variety of scales for color, for color difference, and for white colors. Also, there are different scales for gloss and other geometric attributes of materials.

Complexity of Total Appearance and Limited Applicability of Specific Appearance Scales

Involving, as it does, a potentially infinite variety in both spectral and geometric distributions (to say nothing of varieties in shape, markings, and the like), one can see that total appearance is very complex. It is only feasible with instruments to measure specific attributes of appearance which are important to those who have use for them. These methods, which do exist, have proved to be valid and useful for identifying and controlling product appearance even though they measure only partial, not total appearance.

Appearance measurements are used to provide scientists, engineers, and technologists with quantitative permanent data about important attributes of products. Measurements are needed because the eye, though versatile, cannot assign numbers suitable for records or for quantitative comparisons. Thus, the justifications for appearance measurements are as follows.

1. They assign numbers and thus facilitate communication about appearance.

2. They employ standardized conditions of observation and provide permanent records.

3. They can be selected to have specific observing conditions critical for the product at hand.

4. They can be used in conjunction with computations to derive formulations which are fundamentally more accurate than formulations by skilled artists.

TABLE 2–*Idealized geometric distribution of light for four classes of objects and the major appearance attributes of each.*

Object Class	Idealized Distribution of Light	Dominant Appearance Attribute	Other Appearance Attributes
Opaque non-metals Painted panel Ceremic tile Heavy fabric Pad of paper	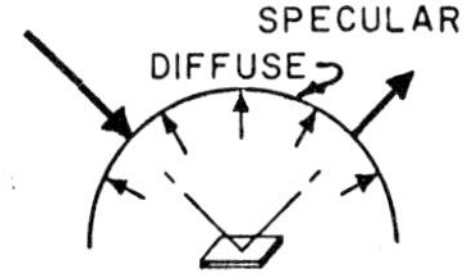	Color (chromaticity and lightness): by diffuse reflection	Gloss: by specular reflection
Opaque metals Auto bumper Brass doorplate	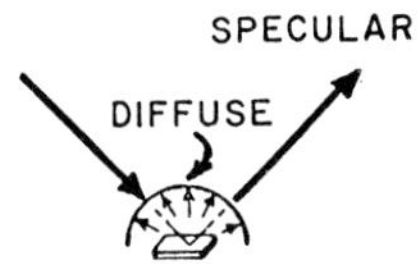	Color (chromaticity and shininess): by specular reflection	Haze or diffuseness: by diffuse reflection
Translucent Plastic light enclosure	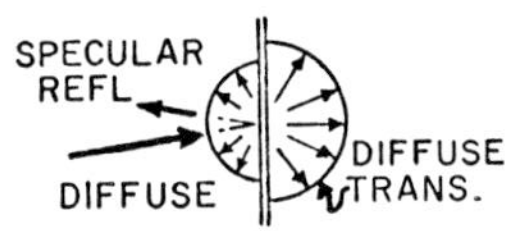	Color (chromaticity and lightness): by diffuse transmission	Gloss: by specular reflection and color by diffuse reflection
Transparent Vegetable oil Sunglass lens	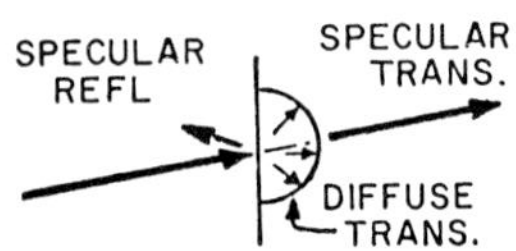	Color (chromaticity and transparency): by specular transmission	Gloss: by specular reflection haze or turbidity: by diffuse transmission

TABLE 3–*ASTM methods for appearance identification of diffusely reflecting materials.*

Attributes	Products and ASTM Committees Involved				
	All Products E-12	Paints D-1	Plastics D-20	Paper D-6 Soap D-12	Ceramics C-21, C-22, C-15
Chromatic Attributes					
Spectrophotometric curves	E 308-66				
CIE color: X,Y,Z,x,y	E 308-66				
L,a,b, surface color					
Munsell color		D 1535-68			
Color difference in L,a,b		D 2244-68			C 609-67(1971)
Color differences in other scales		D 2244-68 D 2616-67			
White colors:					
Whiteness indices	E 313-67				
Yellowness indices	E 313-67		D 1925-70		
Luminous (Green) Reflection Factor	E 97-55			D 3050-72T	C 523-68
Blue Reflection Factor	E 97-55(1971)			D 985-50	
Pigment quality:					
Colored		D 3022-72			
White		D 2745-70			
Geometric Attributes					
Goniophotometric curves	E 167-63(1970)				
Luminous Reflection factor	E 97-55(1971)				C 347-57(1967) C 523-68
Opacity (Hiding power)		D 2805-70		D 589-65(1970)	
Retroreflectance factor		D 1011-52(1970)			
Specular gloss		D 523-67(60°, 20°) D 1471-69(60°)	D 2457-70(60°, 20°, 45°)	D 1223-67(75°) D 1834-65(1970) (20°)	C 346-59(1967)(45°) C 584-71(60°)
Luster					
Distinctiness of image gloss					C 540-67
Sheen		D 523-67(85°)			

TABLE 4—*ASTM methods of appearance identification of metals and light transmitting materials.*

Attributes	Products and ASTM Committees Involved				
	All Products Metals E-12	Resins, Oils, Liquids D-1, D-2 D-23, D-26, E-15	Plastic Sheet, Film D-20	Waxes Polishes, D-21	Other Materials
Chromatic Attributes					
Spectrophotometric curves	E 308-66				
CIE Color: X,Y,Z,x,y	E 308-66				
L,a,b, Object Color		E 450-72T			
Color Difference		E 450-72T			
Yellowness Indices	E 313-67	D 1500-64(1968) (Union) D 1209-69 (Platinum-cobalt) D 1544-68 (Gardner) D 1686-61 (1972) (Platinum-cobalt) D 156-64 (1968) (Saybolt) D 2108-71 (Platinum Cobalt)	D 1925-70		
Geometric Attributes					
Goniophotometric curves	E 166-63 (1970) E 167-63 (1970) (Refl.)				
Diffuse reflection factor	E 429-71				
Reflection haze	E 430-71				
Specular gloss	E 429-71 E 430-71		D 2457-70 (60°, 20°, 45°)	D 1455-64 (60°)	
Distinctness-of-image gloss	E 430-71				
Surface directionality	E 429-71 E 430-71				
Luminous transmission factor			D 1003-61 (1970) D 1494-60 (1969)		
Transmission haze			D 1003-61 (1970)		
Transmission distinctness of image (transparency)			D 1746-70		
Transmission image displacement			D 881-48 (1970) D 637-50 (1970)		

5. They can be used to guide improvement of product quality and saving of money in a variety of ways.

ASTM Achievements in Appearance Attributes Analysis

The American Society for Testing and Materials (ASTM) leads the world in publishing and promoting technical procedures for analyzing the appearance of objects and materials. For many of the products with which ASTM deals, appearance is important. Frequently, the way products look is important because of consumer concerns and preferences for specific appearance attributes or appearance uniformity in the products they buy. There are instances, however, where optical analyses of appearance are useful for the assessment of product performance, for the analysis of ingredients, for studies of processing variables, and for other purposes.

ASTM committees have concerned themselves with measurements of appearance for 40 years or more. ASTM Committee D-1 on Paint, Varnish, Lacquer, and Related Products was probably the first ASTM materials committee to concern itself actively with appearance properties. ASTM D 307 on Spectrophotometry and Description of Color (discontinued, replaced by D 308) and ASTM Test for Specular Gloss (D 523-67) were both issued by Committee D-1 in the 1930's. Other early optical test methods for paints involved hiding power and tinting strength of colored and white pigments, yellowness of oils and resins, and other optical attributes of paints and their ingredients. Many of the older pragmatic tests required only visual comparisons of samples with standards; not physical measurements of samples with instruments for numbers corresponding to product appearance. The present paper is concerned primarily with the more recent quantitative methods of test.

In the 1930's, ASTM Committees D-6 on Paper and Paper Products and D-20 on Plastics worked on measurements of the optical appearance properties of their products. The ASTM Test for Opacity of Paper (D 589-65) was started in the late 1930's.

After World War II, ASTM became involved in the measurement of appearance attributes in many product areas. Then in 1948, ASTM Committee E-12 on Appearance of Materials was formed to work specifically in this one area. This group is now responsible for 12 or more general purpose appearance measurement procedures in the *Annual Book of ASTM Standards.* The following ASTM committees are known to be responsible for ASTM procedures for instrumental appearance attribute analyses, and there are probably others.

Committee E-12 on Appearance of Materials
Committee D-1 on Paint, Varnish, Lacquer, and Related Products
Committee D-20 on Plastics
Committee D-6 on Paper and Paper Products
Committee D-12 on Soaps and Other Detergents

Committee D-13 on Textile Materials
Committee D-21 on Polishes
Committee D-23 on Cellulose and Cellulose Derivatives
Committee D-26 on Halogenated Organic Solvents
Committee C-21 on Ceramic Whitewares and Related Products
Committee C-22 on Porcelain Enamel and Related Ceramic-Metal Systems
Committee C-15 on Manufactured Masonry Units
Committee E-15 on Analysis and Testing of Industrial Chemicals

The actual ASTM methods of tests and recommended practices issued by each of these committees are listed in Table 5.

ASTM published methods of appearance analysis, which require instrumental measurements and are familiar to the author, are listed in numerical order in Table 5, and in Tables 3 and 4 and 6 are divided according to type of product analyzed and the attributes involved. As indicated, Table 3 lists the methods for appearance identification of diffusely reflecting surfaces. This table lists the greatest number of published methods as well as those which enjoy greatest use. It includes methods for finished paints, papers, ceramics, and reflecting plastics. Table 4 lists the methods for metallic and light-transmitting objects and includes a number of test procedures for the yellowness of liquids and the light-transmitting properties of plastic sheets and films. The methods for rating yellowness of liquids and those for light transmitting properties of plastic sheets and films enjoy widespread use.

Table 5 lists four ASTM published documents which do not specify instrumental methods of measurements, but are rather concerned with terminology, standards, and conditions for appearance evaluation: E 179-66, E 259-66, E 284-67, and E 306-71.

Completeness of ASTM's Coverage of Appearance Attribute Analyses

The ASTM procedures identified in this paper constitute the largest group of appearance analysis methods published by any single organization. One can note, however, from the blank spaces in Tables 3 and 4 that there are a number of attributes for which ASTM methods of test applicable to specific products are not yet available. Even in the first (all products) columns, which is in the province of Committee E-12, there are many blanks. Further, by no means are all the appearance attributes which persons might wish to measure identified in Tables 3 and 4.

Roughly, 50 published ASTM methods, involved with the instrumental analysis of appearance of products and materials, are identified. Although the writer is not familiar with the extent to which each of these different methods is employed, he is willing to estimate that no more than 50 percent enjoy wide and general use. Certainly, there are within this list methods such as ASTM D 523-67 and ASTM Test for Haze and Luminous Transmittance of Transparent Plastics

TABLE 5–*ASTM test methods and titles.*

ASTM Methods	Part No., *ASTM Annual Book of Standards*	Titles
C 346-59 (1967)	13	Test for 45° Specular Gloss of Ceramic Materials
C 347-57 (1967)	13	Test for Reflectivity and Coefficient of Scatter of White Porcelain Enamels
C 523-68	14	Test for Light Reflectance of Acoustical Materials by the Integrating Sphere Reflectometer
C 540-67	13	Test for Image Gloss of Porcelain Enamel Surfaces
C 584-71	13	Test for 60° Specular Gloss of Glazed Ceramic Whitewares and Related Products
C 609-67 (1971)	13	Measurement of Small Color Differences Between Ceramic Wall or Floor Tile
D 156-64 (1968)	17, 18	Test for Saybolt Color of Petroleum Products (Saybolt Chronometer Method)
D 523-67	21, 27	Test for Specular Gloss
D 589-65 (1970)	15	Test for Opacity of Paper
D 637-50 (1970)	27	Test for Surface Irregularities of Flat Transparent Plastic Sheets
D 881-48 (1970)	27	Test for Deviation of Line of Sight Through Transparent Plastics
D 985-50 (1969)	15	Test for 45°, 0° Directional Reflectance for Blue Light (Brightness) of Paper
D 1003-61 (1970)	27	Test for Haze and Luminous Transmittance of Transparent Plastics
D 1011-52 (1970)	21	Test for Night Visibility of Traffic Paints
D 1209-69	20,21	Test for Color of Clear Liquids (Platinum-Cobalt Scale)
D 1223-67	15	Test for Specular Gloss of Paper and Paperboard at 75°
D 1455-64 (1971)	22	Test for 60° Specular Gloss of Emulsion Floor Polish
D 1471-69	21	Test for Two-Parameter, 60° Specular Gloss
D 1494-60 (1969)	26	Test for Diffuse Light Transmission Factor of Reinforced Plastics Panels
D 1500-64 (1968)	17,18,29	Test for ASTM Color of Petroleum Products (ASTM Color Scale)
D 1535-68	15,21,30	Specifying Color by the Munsell System
D 1544-68	20,21	Test for Color of Transparent Liquids (Gardner Color Scale)
D 1686-61 (1972)	20	Test for Color of Solid Aromatic Hydrocarbons and Related Materials in the Molten State (Platinum-Cobalt Scale)
D 1746-70	27	Test for Transparency of Plastic Sheeting
D 1834-65 (1970)	15, 18	Test for 20° Specular Gloss of Waxed Paper
D 1925-70	27	Test for Yellowness Index of Plastics

TABLE 5–*ASTM test methods and titles* (Continued).

ASTM Methods	Part No., *ASTM Annual Book of Standards*	Titles
D 2108-71	22	Test for Color of Halogenated Organic Solvents and Their Admixtures (Platinum-Cobalt Scale)
D 2244-68	21,30	Instrumental Evaluation of Color Differences of Opaque Materials
D 2457-70	27	Test for Specular Gloss of Plastic Films (60°, 20°, 45°)
D 2616-67	21	Evaluating Change in Color with a Gray Scale
D 2745-70	20	Test for Instrumental Tinting Strength of White Pigments
D 2805-70	21	Test for Hiding Power of Paints
D 3022-72	21	Test for Color and Strength of Color Pigments by Use of a Miniature Sandmill
D 3050-72T	22	Test for Measuring Soil Removal and Reflectance Retention of Fabrics
E 97-55 (1971)	13,15,30	Test for 45°, 0° Directional Reflectance of Opaque Specimens by Filter Photometry
E 166-63 (1970)	30	Practice for Goniophotometry of Transmitting Objects and Materials
E 167-63 (1970)	30	Practice for Goniophotometry of Reflecting Objects and Materials
E 179-66	30	Practice for Selection of Geometric Conditions for Measurement of Reflectance and Transmittance
E 259-66	15,21,30	Practice for Preparation of Reference White Reflectance Standards
E 284-67	30	Definition of Terms Relating to Appearance of Materials
E 306-71	30	Absolute Calibration of Reflectance Standards
E 308-66	21,30	Practice for Spectrophotometry and Description of Color in CIE 1931 System
E 313-67	21,30	Test for Indexes of Whiteness and Yellowness of Near-White Opaque Materials
E 429-71	30	Measurement and Calculation of Reflecting Characteristics of Metallic Surfaces Using Integrating Sphere Instruments
E 430-71	30	Measurement of Gloss of High Gloss Metal Surfaces Using Abridged Goniophotometer or Goniophotometer
E 450-72T	22	Measurement of Color of Low-Colored Clear Liquids Using the Hunterlab Color Difference Meter

TABLE 6–*Appearance attributes for which standard methods of test are needed, and estimated progress toward realization.*

Steps Toward Realization of Standard Method of Test	Direct Chromatic Attribute Measurements by Tristimulus Colorimetry				Geometric Attributes			
					Gloss			
	Color of Object Surfaces	Color Difference Between Surfaces	Metamerism: Surface-Color Difference Change with Illuminant Change	Color of Objects Other Than Diffusing Surfaces	High Gloss	Luster	Transmission Correlates of Gloss (transparency, haze)	Surface and Film Uniformity Analysis
Select concept for measurement of the attribute	↓	↓	↓	Next Step	↓	↓	↓	Next Step
Select instruments for the measurements	↓	↓	↓		↓	↓	Next Step	
Recommend specific instrumental procedures for calibration, specimen preparation, and measurement	↓	↓	Next Step		Next Step	Next Step		
Document procedure; obtain acceptance by consensus of vote of those interested in the procedure	Next Step	Next Step						

D 1003-61 (1970) which enjoy world-wide use. Both of these methods were originally developed in ASTM, yet their use has now spread so widely that almost everywhere in the world one finds the materials for which they were designed regularly tested and rated by these ASTM procedures.

Perhaps 25 percent of the methods identified in the tables enjoy use in research and development laboratories, but not in the routine analyses of products. Examples of published methods which do not yet enjoy general technical use are ASTM Measurement and Calculation of Reflecting Characteristics of Metallic Surfaces Using Integrating Sphere Instruments (E 429-71) and ASTM Measurement of Gloss of High Gloss Metal Surfaces Using Abridged Goniophotometer or Goniophotometer (E 430-71) for the metallic appearance of metal surfaces. These two methods are new. It will take a period of time for them to be tried and to become established. Another example is ASTM Practice for Spectrophotometry and Description of Color in CIE 1931 System (E 308-66). This method is actually the successor for ASTM D 307, one of the oldest appearance procedures in ASTM books. This method does not enjoy general use in quality analysis of materials because the experimental techniques involved are too complex for use successfully by any but a few highly experienced workers. Spectrophotometry is widely used in chemical analyses, product intercomparisons, and in color formulation. As published, however, ASTM E 308-66 cannot be said to be a recommended practice in wide-spread general use.

Perhaps another 25 percent of the test methods listed enjoy negligible use. Even these methods which are seldom used are frequently referenced as would-be textbooks and papers because of the technical information they contain. Examples of these seldom-used methods are ASTM Practice for Goniophotometry of Transmitting Objects and Materials (E 166-63(1970)) and ASTM Practice for Goniophotometry of Reflecting Objects and Materials (E 167-63(1970)). This instrumental technique enjoys very little use in the assessment of materials because methods of utilizing the results of goniophotometry are not developed. The instruments are rare, so, although goniophotometry is the basic physical method of analyzing the manners in which objects distribute reflected and transmitted light, the standard ASTM procedures and practices for goniophotometry enjoy but little use.

Another ASTM method which enjoys limited use is ASTM Test for Two-Parameter, 60° Specular Gloss (D 1471-69). Here, the reproducible operation of the test method is too difficult to achieve in relation to the value of the information which it yields. Newer test procedures such as those in ASTM E 430-71 can be expected to supplant the technically, rather clumsy method described in ASTM D 1471-69.

Thus, ASTM has made an excellent start on the problem of analyzing appearance attributes of materials by standard methods and procedures. It has accomplished more than any other organization in the world in this area. Still, much needs to be done in preparing procedures where none now exist. The utility of under-utilized procedures needs to be improved.

Major Unmet Needs and Suggested ASTM Program for the Appearance Analysis of Materials

Before any instrumental method of appearance analysis can be standardized, several developments must be completed.

1. A concept or plan must be available to measure the attribute in question.
2. Suitable instruments must be available to make the measurement.
3. Investigators must work with instruments and specimens of the products to be tested, then recommend procedures for instrumental calibration, specimen preparation, and measurement techniques.
4. These procedures must be documented and accepted by a concensus of those having an economic interest in the proposed procedure.

In the following paragraphs, some unmet needs for testing chromatic attributes and geometric attributes of appearances of materials are described. These are listed in Table 6, together with estimates of the progress already made toward their realization. Not considered in the present study are the many opportunities which exist for adapting specific methods of measurement to meet the needs of the specific product technologies for improved analyses of appearance attributes. Only general purpose methods of testing appearance are considered in this section.

Unmet Needs for Chromatic Attribute Analysis

Simple Reproducible Method for Surface-Color Measurement—A method of color measurement is urgently needed which is simple enough for operation by the usual lab technician and, nevertheless, yields results reproducible from one laboratory to another. Such a method to be generally satisfactory for use in the paint, paper, textile, plastics, and other industries should also be readily reproducible concerning the magnitude of the average commercial color tolerance. Only recently have instruments been developed which are able to achieve this accuracy when used properly and, nevertheless, have the simplicity and ruggedness for operation by average laboratory technicians.

There are actually two types of instruments now available which are able to achieve the needed reproducible, rapid surface-color measurements. First are the photoelectric tristimulus colorimeters which now have the accuracy of spectral response required for accuracy in color and color difference measurement. Billmeyer, and Hunter and Gibson have reported on the accuracy of these instruments. Second are the abridged spectrophotometers which have become simpler to keep in calibration and have been combined with built-in computers so that the necessary tristimulus color values are obtained automatically.

Billmeyer has reported on the accuracy of these instruments. Thus, methods of surface-color measurement by both of these instruments are now ready for laboratory experimentation as identified by Step 3. Step 4 in the preparation of the ASTM Method in writing would then follow and there seems now to be no obstacle to the successful realization of practical methods of surface-color measurement.

A project now under way in ASTM Committee C-22 on Porcelain Enamel and Related Ceramic-Metal Systems is worthy of mention in connection with this need for a method of surface-color measurement. The project is designed to complete work on Hunter's proposal made in 1962 for tristimulus colorimeter diagnostic standards which will establish when color measuring instruments have the reproducibility and spectral accuracy required. The program is actually aimed toward the preparation of a general purpose set of diagnostic standards to be used in assessing the accuracy and reproducibility of surface-color measuring instruments.

Methods for Color Difference—A second need is related to the first and involves methods for the measurement of color difference. Actually an ASTM method is already on the ASTM books (ASTM Instrumental Evaluation of Color Differences of Opaque Materials (D 2244-68)), which identifies seven different measurement scales available for use in analyses of color differences. As presently written, ASTM D 2244-68 identifies chiefly the various color-difference scales in terms of tristimulus values. It is not concerned with instrument calibration or accuracy. When a reproducible, generally acceptable method for the measurement of surface color is developed to meet the first need, it can be anticipated that the corresponding method of color difference measurement will probably be selected for ASTM attention. The primary requirement is, as with the first need, that standard methods for calibration of instruments and assurance of reproducibility from one to another be established and used.

Metamerism—Associated with the need for color difference measurements between surfaces is a requirement for an extension of the adopted procedure so that it can be used to measure degree of metamerism. Metamerism can be described as the increase or change in color difference between two similarly colored surfaces when the illuminant on them is changed. Here, it can be seen in Table 6, simple instrumental procedures are not yet generally available. However, the need exists, and as colorimeters and spectrophotometers improve in accuracy and flexibility, it can be expected that devices will become available which can measure color differences in a variety of illuminants.

Actually, the wide-spread use of 16-filter abridged spectrophotometers in the area of color measurement can be expected to hasten progress toward agreement on measurement of metamerism. These filter abridged spectrophotometers are readily adaptable to metamerism evaluation; whereas the simpler tristimulus instruments have not yet been so modified.

Measurement of Object Colors for Other Than Diffusing Surfaces—The fourth, and last, unmet need in the area of chromatic scales is for reproducible methods to measure colors of objects other than diffusely reflecting surfaces. By reference to Table 6, it can be seen that here the practical procedures for measurement are not yet suggested. In fact, neither the instruments, nor the measurement scales most suitable to this type of specimen are as yet identified for certainty. Proposals for color scales have been made and some trials of them have been carried out, but progress toward meeting this last unmet requirement is definitely behind that in the surface-color area effort.

Needs in the Geometric Attribute Area

High Gloss Method for Non-Metal Surfaces—The first need in the geometric area is for a convenient, readily reproducible method for high gloss measurement. The primary obstacle to success in this type of measurement is the absence of techniques for readily making reproducible measurements of high gloss. Procedures have been proposed, and it has been established that with test methods such as the one specifically intended for metal surfaces, and identified in ASTM E 430-71, significant differences in high gloss can readily be measured. However, the instrumental techniques required for successful measurement of high gloss differences by this method require extreme care in the geometric orientation of the instrument with respect to the surface under test. However, progress is being made in the development of this type of measurement.

Luster—Again in the gloss area, there exist several needs for standardized reproducible methods of luster measurement. Luster, or the recognition of gloss as a contrast between shiny areas of surfaces and their surroundings, is an important criterion in textile, plastic fabric, and diffuse metal surface appearance analysis. Instrumental techniques for this are readily available and have been proven practical, but the pressure has never been great enough in this area to bring about selection of specific test procedures for any of the considerable number of products for which luster is important.

Transmission Correlates of Gloss—The third of the geometric attributes for which methods are needed are transmission correlates of gloss, such as transparency, haze, and the like. Actually, there exists a well-established and widely-used method for transmission haze of plastic films. There is also a plastics-film method for distinctness of transmitted image. Concepts for the other attributes of transmission gloss correspond quite simply to the concepts for reflection gloss. Here the needs for the methods of measurement have not yet been adequately identified. For this reason, work to bring the test methods to realization has not been carried out.

Uniformity Analysis—The fourth, and last, of the basic needs for geometric attribute measurement involves surface and film uniformity analysis. These uniformity analyses would be used to measure appearance attributes such as texture, sharpness in printing, legibility, and perhaps mottle printability and the like. Scanning methods will be essential to assess surfaces for optical uniformity over the area in view. In this area it is necessary to develop concepts of how surface uniformity may be quantified so as to get numbers representing texture, or print sharpness, or mottle. There would seem to be major opportunities for the creation of instrumentation and useful methods of testing in this area.

Conclusion

Although the ASTM is well ahead of the rest of the world in the development of published methods for measurement of appearance attributes of materials, much remains to be done. Not only are new and better methods of appearance analysis needed, but publicity for wider use of the methods already prepared is also required. In the United States, ASTM leads the way while other organizations such as The American National Standards Institute (ANSI), The Technical Association of the Pulp and Paper Industry (TAPPI), and The American Association of Textile Chemists and Colorists (AATCC) follow the lead of the ASTM in the promotion and use of such standards. Use of ASTM procedures is spreading to the international sphere. Through ANSI, ASTM methods are being promoted and, in many cases, adopted by the International Standards Organization (ISO). For the work foreseen in the present paper, ASTM and other groups must develop, prove, and then publicize the practicability of various consensus methods for the measurement of appearance attributes.

Bibliography

Hardy, A. C., *Handbook of Colorimetry,* Massachusetts Institute of Technology Press, Cambridge, Mass., 1936.

Annual Book of ASTM Standards, American Society for Testing and Materials, Philadelphia, Pa.

Billmeyer, F. W., Jr., *Applied Optics,* Vol. 8, April 1969, p. 775.

Hunter and Gibson, "Improvement of the Accuracy of Photoelectric Tristimulus Colorimeters," *Color Engineering,* March-April 1969.

Hunter, R. S., "Tests for the Uniformity of 45° 0° Reflectometers," *Journal of the Optical Society of America,* March 1963.

C. J. Abend [1]

Product Appearance as Communication

REFERENCE: Abend, C. J., **"Product Appearance as Communication,"** *Sensory Evaluation of Appearance of Materials, STP 545,* American Society for Testing and Materials, 1973, pp. 35-53.

ABSTRACT: To those in the world of designed objects, most specifically industrial design, it soon becomes evident that the development of form, creation of appearance, and selection of materials, result in product communication. An inherent message always exists and it may be composed consciously or subconsciously; furthermore, it is received and understood without written or verbal intervention and is instantaneous with respect to the impression it evokes. Such responses are subjective but are similar in interpretation within a specific population. The meaning of the communicated product message can create *immediate bias* or *almost unshakeable beliefs* with respect to the product observed; frequently, to the extent that it can overshadow intellectual or rational considerations. Automotive design is a good example.

Where communication is negative, it can produce the familiar dichotomy expressed as the complaint, "I know it's good, but I just don't like it." Rejection or acceptance, it would appear, has much to do with the visually-perceived qualities of the communication established between product and observer. In product design, such communicated attributes as credibility, convenience, prestige, value, usefulness, genuineness, and even masculinity or feminity are largely dependent upon a number of factors not the least of which is the characteristic appearance of materials used in the design context. The question is examined as to why man-made objects attract or repel. Some probable explanations are considered in this paper. These are believed to be correlations that exist between psychological and social factors as they are aesthetically expressed and visually perceived.

It appears likely that all products, as a result of their aesthetic properties, conditioned by visual associations and appearance of materials, influence subjective response in favorable or unfavorable ways. This indicates the presence of communication via a design language, the semantics of which requires more explicit definitions. The groundwork for a vocabulary is suggested, a method for appearance rating is proposed, and areas for future research are identified.

KEY WORDS: senses, communicating, perception, design, aesthetics

[1] Vice president, Industrial Design, SCM Corporation, Syracuse, N. Y. 13203.

Appearance plays many roles. R. S. Hunter, in his paper, "Appearance Attributes of Metallic Surfaces," [*1*] [2] describes one aspect,

> in finishing metals, the mill technologist does not think in terms of extinction coefficients, spectrophotometrics curves or goniophotometric curves. He thinks in terms of adjustments he must make to the finishing process, the ingredients of the equipment to bring about *the appearance* which his customer desires.

It is apparent that, for the technician, the scientist, or the researcher, appearance attributes have different qualities and dimensions. For the designer, these qualities go beyond measurement which relates only to structural or physical properties. To the designer, product appearance holds the key to communication.

In the definition of its scope, ASTM Committee E-18 on Sensory Evaluation of Materials in Products states one of its major objectives as being "The promotion of knowledge, stimulation of research, and the development of principles and recommended practice for sensory evaluation (including discrimination and preference) of materials and products." The significant point for designers, researchers, and industry concerns the matter of discrimination and preference. It is this aspect which bears a relationship to appearance as communication. Although a great deal is understood about the technical standards which control appearance, its aesthetic meaning is still illusive and goes beyond physical parameters.

It is my contention that discrimination and preference are regulated by appearance qualities. I concur wholeheartedly with ASTM and Committee E-18 in their interest to consider additional aspects of appearance study, and I recommend focus on industrial design as an area which holds much promise.

As clarification to the reader, where the words "design" or "industrial design" are used, it is meant as the total outcome of a creative and premeditated process of development. Appearance, thus, represents the outer manifestation of configuration, selection of materials, human factors, as well as manufacturing, engineering, and cost considerations.

Product Appearance as Communication

Appearance as communication raises some aspect of novelty by suggesting that man-made objects have the power of "speaking to us" and of transmitting a message. Simplistic as this may seem, it is my contention that this happens when we perceive objects. A message is contained and conveyed through the media of the appearance qualities of the object which are an inseparable part of its design. These elements deliver their particular meanings which seem to be comprehended by specific populations. The relationships between appearance communi-

[2] The italic numbers in brackets refer the list of references appended to this paper.

cation and sensory perception is one which requires further psychological and sociological study to lay the groundwork for interpretation guidance and application.

Where the word communication is used, it is generally regarded to mean the transmission of written or verbal information. Such communication is sequential in nature; data bits are received and linked in accordance with a learned schema; written or spoken code represents vicarious values and experiences. The word "pain" for example, stands for a condition which becomes much less abstract through actual sensation. A picture illustrating pain would come closer to communicating this meaning and evoking the expected response. Written and verbal communication have limitations because they use codes that are abstract and must be acquired. A more total presentation of meaning occurs in painting and sculpture [*2*], in which an idea is communicated without verbal intervention. The expressive use of human form such as Rodin's "The Thinker" is so evident that, regardless of the language of the observer, little more has to be said about the experience of pondering and deliberation. The entire story content is delivered to us at once. I believe product design, as a similar kind of configurational expression, is no less capable of delivering meaningful ideas. Design ideas are transferred by relying similarly on premeditated and aesthetic cues.

These aesthetic values are space, volume, proportion, scale and texture, etc. The difference between sculpture and a product is that expectation of expression occurs in the former; communication takes place in both, but in the product it is not intellectualized, and thus thought to be absent. Who could believe that such objects as tables and chairs possess meanings? Nevertheless, we know that a message is received because consensus of discrimination and preference usually exists and can be measured. Insofar as industrial designers try to understand and plan its human consequences, the design of a product is a concern with communication. Design characteristics carry significant cues for human behavior. Most designers intuitively select the conditions for response; what is absent is a rationale for determining the meaning evoked by a specific design.

The process of product communication can be considered ephemeral and can go unrecognized by both designer and his audience. Product designs emerge as a solution-oriented creation, conditioned by both intuitive and rational judgments and governed by physical and economic limitations; yet, in the end, their final form seems to defy explanations. The challenge of "Why did you do it like this?" are often painful questions put to the designer and, similarly, "Tell me *exactly* why you don't like it" is equally perplexing to the observer. The answer, in both cases, may lie in the quality of the message content itself. Upon this is dependent the rapport between form-giver and perceiver.

This visual language is transmitted via appearance and the materials used.

Thus, to relate visually perceived attributes to product appearance requires a vocabulary which is not yet defined. The complexity of this task is self-evident; as in any language, there are many ways of saying things. This is dependent upon the skill of the designer. It is within his power to say things more practically, poetically, or more convincingly, than others—or to say them in ways that rankle and produce a negative response.

Product appearance is a general description of the intelligence and sophistication which produced it; it imparts information relative to manual dexterity, comprehension, beliefs, psychological needs and, sometimes, even type of government. R. S. Latham [*3*] says

> All of these things are read out of objects every day by the unskilled layman. It is the silent language of the senses. It occurs at the unspoken emotional level and judgments are formed, trains of logic instigated, and action taken on the basis of this language. This is the first way a human being accumulates the information necessary to make judgments.

Visual Perception—Key to Communication

To examine the idea of appearance communication we must consider the related nature of visual perception which begins in infancy and is governed by biological human development and experience. Mussen et al [*4*] report revealing findings:

> Work by neuro-physiologists indicates that the visual areas of the cortex are responsive to contoured edges in particular spatial orientations. This suggests that the longer attention to the stimula with contours (by infants) is not based on learning but is the result of biological characteristics of the nervous system. This tendency to look at contour will leave the infant to focus his attention on his mother's eyes because of their inherent black/white contrast.

The answers to adult response may be found in infancy which may offer clues about reaction to usual stimuli. What is the degree to which inherent biological responses rather than learned responses prevail in their effect on visual perception. Experiments have indicated, for example, that infants look longer at more complex stimuli as they grow older. Additionally, it is reported that contrast and movement are not the *only* governors of the infant's attention. Later on, there are other influences, primarily the effect of *meaning* and *familiarity of the stimuli,* and there are attentional preferences for stimuli which supersede infant interest in contrast and movement. On the aspect of the attentiveness, the relation of the stimulus to an acquired "schema" becomes a new determinant of attention. (Schema is a condition which stands for some internal representation of an experience—it can also be an idea or event.) A child's memory of its mother's face can be a schema and it will relate to patterns or pictures to the degree that they reveal some correspondence.

I am prepared to accept the deduction that *attention, discrimination, and aesthetic preference must be compatible to schema which is biologically conditioned.* This may vary among individuals which might explain individual tastes; nevertheless, there appears to be such a thing as aesthetic consensus. The sensory and communicative attributes of appearance will depend upon further inquiries into its physiological and psychological roots. One such area is research having to do with pleasure centers in the brain. Experiments on laboratory animals suggest new implications. In implanting electrodes into specific areas of the brain, pleasure sensations were reproduced by other than the normal stimula. To quote researcher, James Olds[5],

> Why is the electrical stimulation so rewarding? We are currently exploring this question working on the hypothesis that brain stimulation in these regions must excite some of the nerve cells that would be excited by satisfaction of the basic drive—hunger, sex, thirst, etc. We have looked to see whether some parts of the reward system of the brain are specialized; that is, there may be one part for the hunger drive and another part for the sex drive, etc. . . . Our present tentative conclusion is that emotional and motivational mechanisms can indeed be localized in the brain; that certain portions of the brain are sensitive to each of the basic drives. Strong electrical stimulation of these areas seems to be even more satisfying than the usual rewards of food, etc.

Olds suggests that research conclusions are likely to be generalized eventually to human beings. We are then left to speculate; Does visual perception, such as in product appearance, excite electrical impulses in the brain to produce pain or pleasure? When we exercise appearance discrimination or preference, are we being regulated by hedonic biological recognition of stimuli which are to be sought or avoided? We are left to speculate as to the degree of influence that such visual gratification has in the appearance communication process itself. The old adage that "beauty is in the eye of the beholder" does not seem too outlandish after all.

Approaching an Appearance Vocabulary

A simple analysis of visual vocabulary might begin by isolating two related components. One is aesthetic (shape, contour, line proportion, and texture) and the other is associative. Shape and contour are already known to function as information in signs and symbols; similarly, other aesthetic properties also contribute to meanings. These could be derived from the aesthetics of forms in nature, as well as some of the biological preferences previously mentioned. The component of association is developed by social and personal experience with materials. Together, these two factors establish meanings which could be considered as the basis for an appearance vocabulary.

Sensory experience with materials can form associations which may be transferred such as when used in product appearance. An example of appearance association might be the mood of placidity and fluidity created by the observation of a quiet lake; correspondingly, as the texture, turbidity, and color of the same body of water change under a threatening storm, the associative mood also changes. Thus, a material association is established; yet, the same material with altered texture or color can convey different information. If we respond to such a context, then it must be on the basis of comprehending some fundamental aspect of appearance vocabulary. Researchers cannot yet offer laboratory data to prove that such a vocabulary becomes psychologically imprinted; nevertheless, empirical observations suggest that associative qualities (such as serenity or threat in the case stated) are transferred ideas along with material appearance when it is reproduced in another context. For example, we are familiar with the warmth and security which the infant attaches to soft materials like blankets. Is this inclination forgotten or is it still active in adult behavior in the selection of clothing and other goods where there will be tactile contact? Consider stone and the coldness and finality we associate with say a gravestone marker. Both, association and (aesthetics) shape, play a part here. The permanency, solidity, and massiveness of stone, however, can be transferred without conveying finality merely by altering aesthetics. This occurs in architecture wherein the use of stone expresses lastingness. Our impressions of the gravestone can also be further changed if we substitute a different material. If the marker were constructed of plastic, fur, or sponge, it would conflict with the associative component of this object and would likely be rejected.

Our further understanding of appearance vocabulary is helped by inferences defined by its structure. For example, glass has some of the smooth and transparent characteristics as water; is it possible that glass possesses associations with that serene and placid lake we spoke of? Does the popularity of glass as a container for liquids have something to do with the fact that water is clear and liquid (and was once believed to be potable)?

If this sounds too esoteric, it may be because it is. Is there better evidence? I offer the suspicion that basic sensory experiences which occur by contact with materials in nature form a strong schema for aesthetic and associative values; it is these to which we make subconscious reference even when we encounter them in products. A material which supports this view is wood—a friendly material which no one seems to dislike. To learn why, we might begin by considering man's experience with wood. It was one of the first materials with which he interacted; it lent itself easily to shape and form by his own hand to meet his basic needs. Wood may remind us of a chair, boat, house, or literally thousands of sensory experiences all of which have had agreeable and "warm" associations. For this reason, we frequently see even fake wood being used incongrously as decorative touches in products in order to evoke these very responses.

In order to provoke further thinking along the lines of a possible vocabulary,

I offer a simple and unscientific start towards a generic classification of material characteristics (see Table 1). These descriptive words can be used to classify appearance by texture, structure, or state (the full technical parameters of material definition are obviously not met). The purpose of this exercise is to select any combination of texture, structure, or state to see if one can recall a specific material which can be described by these factors. To start off, let me suggest a porous/homogenous/dense material which might be described as a sponge. Are there aesthetic or associative values that these two materials possess in common? If the sponge lost its flexibility and were hardened into shape, would it resemble concrete? Would it bother you to consider the possibility of using sponges as a building material? Similarly, would it concern you to use a "soft" concrete block to soap down your car?

What is it about these material characteristics which is being communicated? They are all vested with associative values. Can we detect any common visual denominators which suggest an inherent and transferrable vocabulary? Are there relationships which evoke similar responses? If so, then we may be able to isolate those aspects which contain universal meanings. There are more sophisticated approaches, but if we can identify a few reproducible qualities, we are on the threshold of establishing an appearance vocabulary.

As to the possibilities of appearance code, I find it interesting that, whereas appearance is visually perceived, it also relies heavily on other sensory experience. In my opinion, kinesthetic and tactile experience plays a special product role; I believe this is so because of the transfer of associations which become visually reinforced. A piece of ice or glowing coal no longer has to be touched to be believed. Hundreds of tactile learning experiences are established in infancy in which the child literally tastes his way through his environment; it is likely that such experiences are not forgotten. When one observes barbed wire,

TABLE 1–*Appearance description of materials.*[a]

Texture	Structure	State
smooth	loose	pliable
porous	connected	hard
fibrous	compacted	stiff
reflective	opaque	brittle
striated	translucent	flexible
hairy	cellular	viscous
soft	granulated	watery
absorbent	crystalline	dense
rough	homogenous	resilient
textured		powdery

[a] The basic description of materials is shown classified by appearance. There are many possible combinations of appearance qualities which can create a similar subjective response.

the communication is also inescapable—"Don't touch!" The response here is primarily tactile but is coded as material and shape. Change the material to "barbed spaghetti" and it is not likely to evoke anything but a smile.

The entire area of appearance factors continues present interest because its vocabulary is largely unchartered. This unchartered area offers new ground for research by behavioral scientists, sociologists, and market researchers. The non-verbal language of appearance is capable of definition when deeper inquiries produce agreed-upon and reproducible meanings.

Syntax and Forms of Non-Verbal Communication

If configuration is the handwriting of the designer, then such correspondence must be governed by a non-verbal syntax. We are familiar with non-verbal communication in such forms as symbols and pictographs which are conceivably understood as the visual equivalent of words and slogans; they convey only limited ideas. In products, appearance-syntax employs other elements. The relative size of an object, its relationship to other components, linear definition, texture, and so forth, are the elements with which the non-verbal product "sentence" is composed. These identify the subject and main idea, as well as display the visual adjectives by which the content of the message is communicated. What is said is the function of syntax structure; how it is said is the quality of individual style.

There are other forms of non-verbal communication such as gesture and facial expression, and such linguistics have sometimes been carried over into product appearance. We can frequently find similarity to faces or animals whereby the object is "read" by its physiognomy. In the recent past, many industrial age products were treated with applied ornament such as the flowered and embellished cast-iron radiators. These products, borrowed directly from nature were, perhaps, a naive form of associative transfer; nevertheless, imitative devices are still seen today and "jet styling" and air-foil shapes are merely forms borrowed from super products such as aircraft.

In many products, it is not too difficult to identify associations with smoothly-contoured surfaces which resemble the female anatomy. The toothy grin of the old Cadillac bumper, as well as the rear-view facial expression of the Volkswagon are both in the category of such borrowings. Similarly, some of the smaller consumer products take on the disguised characteristics of animals which may appear threatening, reassuring, or cute. Such practice is sometimes deliberate, but it points out the pervasiveness of transferred associations. Along with such transferrence, have also come some ideas. Ruesch and Kees[*6*] take note of the special non-verbal communication of objects.

> Object language, because of its time and enduring qualities, plays an enormous role in archeology, anthropology, and history. Until the discovery of the first written documents to come down to us, the only

enduring traces we had of the remote past were those that survived in the form of objects and buildings. Tools and weapons were known as early as the stone age and the fact that material articles almost always carry either implicit or explicit instructions with them, makes it possible to reconstruct events from prehistoric times, even though we lack knowledge of the verbal language of a particular period.

To paraphrase the authors, objects convey information just as the spoken language; objects possess information coded in design and materials which have survived for centuries. In our accumulative knowledge of the evolution of the earth, man and society have been reconstructed from appearance information coded in object language. Ruesch and Kees make another *salient* observation.

> In linguistics, the field of syntax is given over to the study of mutual relationships of verbal signs to each other. A corresponding relationship in object language is expressed with a combination of materials, surface, structure, color, and shape to produce an object that embodies the functions of noun, adjective, verb, and adverb all in one. Finally, the sequences of sentences leading to the expression of an idea are achieved in object language through the arrangements of several articles (components) in space; the idea that is then expressed might be called a theme.

My contentions are that appearance syntax is built upon associative sensory experience, symbolism, imagery of schema, human expression, and gesture, all of which are structured by the aesthetic configuration. Figure 1 depicts a designer's conceptualization of the communication sequence from object to observer. Each "lens" modifies how the appearance information is treated—and here it might be said that beauty is in the eye of the beholder.

Object and Information—An Illustrative Example

An object which most exemplifies appearance as communication is the hand ax. I have chosen this object because of its simple form and because it is a well-recognized tool. It represents a configuration which was not "designed" but has evolved slowly and which occurs repeatedly in various civilizations. In referring to the hand ax, illustrated in Fig. 2, I would like to examine those appearance elements which make up its design and, which, create a statement about its use. Let us look at the form of the head.

1. It is sharp at one end indicating it is a blade and can cut or penetrate. The width of the blade infers, not only that it is a working surface, but the size of the work possible; the position of the head, relative to the line of the handle, establishes the direction of work. The naked head and its edge are direct about its function because it is exposed, thus, identifies an aspect of hazard; it does not encourage one to grasp this object by the blade.

2. Another form factor is the pointed and wedge shape of the head which is directional and arrow-like in nature; this is a further visual clue with respect to

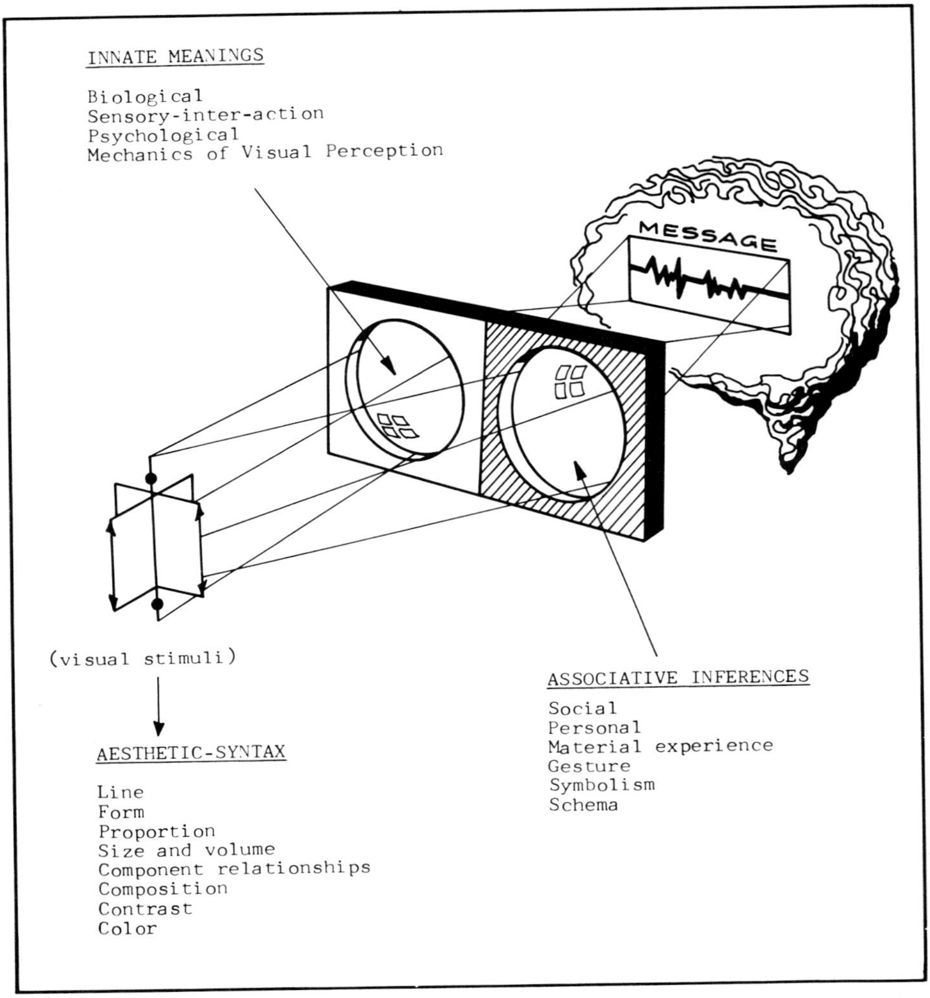

FIG. 1—*Conceptualization of communication sequence.*

direction of work. The back of the head is blunt which reveals thickness and heft; massiveness, and potential inertia are made visible. The head, composed of metal, probably iron or steel, reveals a characteristic metal surface denoting solidity, strength, weight, and denseness. A metal head further suggests that it has the ability to create and withstand impact.

3. Now, look at the handle. To begin with, it is essentially a stick or lever; the inference is that it is to be hand-held and is something to beat with, or to

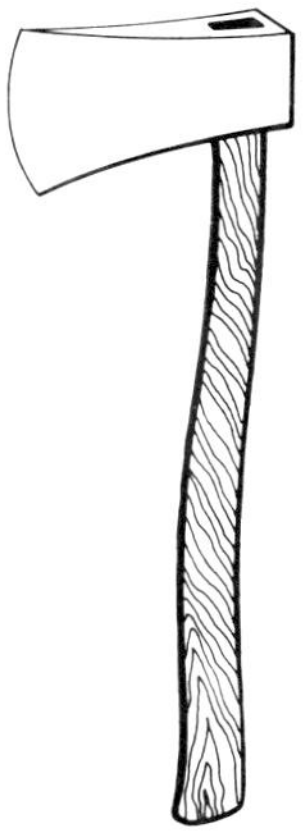

FIG. 2–*AXE–illustrative example of communication.*

wield. The material is wood; this is familiar, and should be agreeable to the touch and inviting the possibility of grasp. The diameter of the handle and the slightly curved section near the bottom, locates an area for grip. This stick, however, can be held anywhere along its surface, and this possibility is shown by its smoothness and length. The fact that it is wood indicates that it may be resilient and perhaps absorb shock. Furthermore, the length of the stick, (about the size of a man's extended arm) suggests that similarly it may be used to swing or strike. Because of the heavy attached head, it is not likely that it should leave the hand; it is evident that it should be restrained.

These are some of the visual clues which I see generated by configuration. Following are further assumptions regarding the combination of the two elements–head and handle. In this respect, they are beautifully articulated in that they compliment the idea of union. The most obvious quality is the apparent tightness of wedge into a split shaft; devised with clear intent, this mating must be contrived for a purpose in which both elements show a permanent relationship to one another. This reasoning is confirmed by the top-heaviness of the blade which suggests that, if lifted, its regulated position is to swing down with respect to gravity. The mass at the end of the stick identifies the advantage of inertia. The ax is its own instruction manual.

This interpretation can be challenged as rationalization after the fact, yet everything about the appearance of the ax seems self-evident. This is because its design is an outgrowth of these very factors. All products possess inherent information, but perhaps not quite as successfully as the ax. This is why I believe that products that communicate well generally survive and those that do not, fail.

A control test we might employ to check appearance communication is to make slight alterations to the ax design and see if this changes the impression of what it communicates to us. Figure 3 is such an experiment in that materials remain unchanged, but only configuration is altered. In Illustration A, the orientation of the head is reversed which strikes most people as odd or frustrating. Illustration B shows the blade position changed to the center of the lever. This ax can still be used but presents a dilemma. In Illustration C, we employ a split handle at the head which forks out into two distinct grips (perhaps this is an improvement as it suggests a two-handed operation). Illustration D, alters the design by means of a change in scale; the size of the tiny blade now seems to have lost all of its advantage of mass and looks inaffective and peculiar, which it is. (The reason for this is similar to why toys look childish to adults—because their appearance is exaggerated and out of scale. This causes the idea to be either over-stated or under-stated. What is being communicated is the fact that they are not meant to be taken seriously but rather as cartoons of the real world.) In the last illustration, E, we have kept proportion and material the same, but changed the shape of the head and handle which is now square. Tactile experience is evoked and one can almost feel the discomfort in this grip; at the same time, the object is no longer an ax. It is something else, perhaps a sledge to be used for breaking rock. With alteration of design, we have altered the information.

Carrying our experiment one step further, in Fig. 4, we have retained configuration but varied only materials. Some of these get to be ridiculous. How do these designs strike you? (Communicate to you?) Analyze your response and try to identify what it is in the message you receive which makes you tolerant or hostile to the appearance.

Illustration A shows a design composed of a solid rubber handle attached to a clear glass blade. Illustration B shows a design of a clay handle which is apparently driven through a wedge of Swiss cheese. (This is what designers call a delicious solution.) Illustration C merely reverses the material; the blade is now

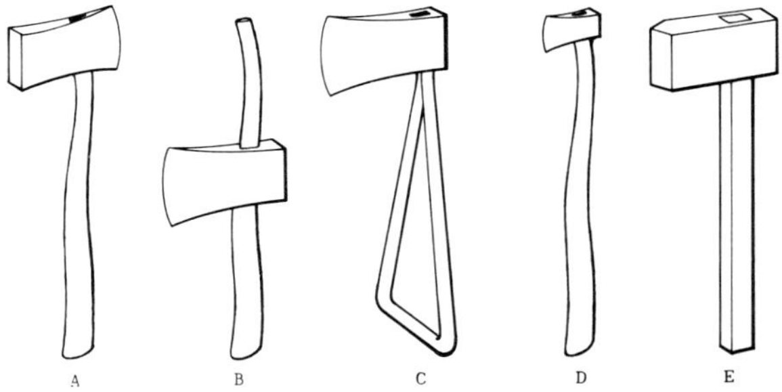

FIG. 3—*Alterations in proportion.*

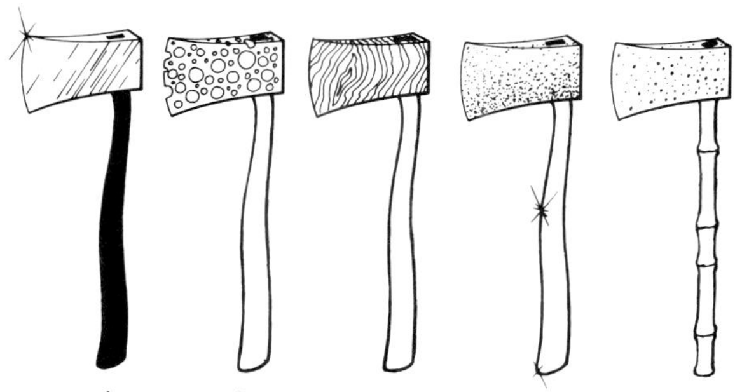

FIG. 4–*Alterations in material.*

made of wood and the handle is made of steel. Illustration D depicts the handle made of plastic (ordinary polystyrene), and the blade made of granulated sugar. Illustration E depicts the handle made of bamboo and the blade of cast concrete.

With these illustrations, I conclude this experiment aimed at provoking a personal response. By means of design alteration, and even the use of nonsense situations, it has served to illustrate some aspects of appearance communication. Whether objects say clean or dirty, cool or warm, hard or soft, up or down, is dependent upon the qualities displayed by materials and design. The ax is not unique; similar appearance factors are intrinsic in more sophisticated products and they communicate with varying degrees of success.

Rating Appearance Communication

Let us consider a formula by which communication effectiveness in products might be judged. The ingredient of good product design is that it shows evidence of clearly satisfying two conditions. These are need (N) and desirability (D). If these values, independently or combined, lead to the threshold of action (or acquisition consideration), then it can be said that positive communication has been established. The relative importance of N and D vary according to type of product. Need is defined as the sense of a basic functional requirement apart from such considerations as, "would like to possess" or "sometimes useful." Luxury items have low need values but high desirability values. Needs can be identified by responses to such questions as "Do I have a problem that must be solved?" "Will this product solve it?" "Can I do without it?" Need as regards a specific product could be weighted relative to (*a*) function or service to be performed, (*b*) special features, and (*c*) requirement (utility or necessity).

Desirability, in my definition, means the over-all design attributes which the product conveys or gratifies. It is everything but need. D stands for a number of discrete qualities which can be possessed by a specific product; these are explained and contribute to the accumulative value of D. The following are my terms with product examples for clarification.

Desirability Is Composed of–

1. Fv (Face Validity)–The visual credibility of the product: ability to do the job and to command belief in service value or price.

   Example: gas-powered chain saw, computer, wood-working tools, microscope

2. Sc (Social Coding)–This represents recognition of group-endorsed values, status, prestige, class distinction, etc; these may either be positive or negative.

   Example: automobiles, jewelry, clothing

3. O (Operation)–The degree to which the application, use and function of the product is expressed and understood.

   Example: ax, bicycle

4. Pa (Possessive Appeal)–Play value, enjoyment or fun of use; pride of ownership, pleasure principle.

   Example: watches, toys, boats

5. Pi (Personal Identity)–Coveted aspirations, personal meanings and motivations, special virtues which the object is felt to bestow on the owner.

   Example: antiques, souvenirs, crafts objects, furniture, jewelry

6. Sy (Sensory)–This quality offers a high degree of sensory satisfaction to the user. Such products produce agreeable tactile or kinesthetic experiences, although not limited to these senses.

   Example: skis, golf clubs, musical instruments, guns

$$D \text{ is the sum of } (Fv + Sc + O + Pa + Pi + Sy)$$

Thus, the Communication Value $= N + D$

or

$$Cv = N + D$$

The term motivation (M) needs also to be considered inasmuch as this acts as a modifying factor on the $N + D$ stimulus. Lack of product availability or high cost creates a disinterested response or essentially a message which will be ignored. A case in point might be a $500 000 robot programmed to set the table and clear the dishes. No doubt, that in American culture such a product might evoke need and desirability values of high degree; unfortunately, price and limited quantity suggest that this is not to be taken seriously. Another example might be the case of a person in an underdeveloped country needing a large farm cultivator. Availability here, as a result of distribution and cost, makes this product unattainable despite the fact that N and D may be very high. Motivation may, thus, be diminished by availability and cost, but also by such factors as amount of search necessary to find the product, lack of parts, service, or complex instruction. Motivation, by this definition, represents those conditions which add to or reduce the effective value of N plus D. It is an obvious deduction that where need and desirability are established and where motivation can be made high, a potential area for market exists. Entering the motivation aspect into the equation, we can now develop a formula for market stimulus value.

A simple equation is suggested to represent the market stimulus value (MSV) of a product design. Our equation reads:

$$MSV = (N + D)\ (\pm M)$$

Some general observations are to be made. The magnitude of Cv (Communicative Value) is the additive result of two stimuli, need and desirability. Where need is high and desirability low, a high magnitude of the communicative value can still be achieved.

This rating method is workable only to the extent to which we can develop proportionately accurate scaling values for N and D. The two components, however, should be equally weighted, but the numerical values assigned to each element can be based on criteria to be established empirically. The factor, M, might range between an assigned value of ± 3. It can be seen that small adjustments to M have significant effect on MSV. MSV is applied only to the applicable spectrum of the market. That is to say, it would be pointless to attempt to rate the MSV of a milling machine against the response of, say, taxi drivers.

It is not likely that appearance communication will ever be exactly rated. We can, however, establish some basic rules for judging the effectiveness of an appearance statement and a means that substitutes rationale for subjective opinionation. The formula $MSV = (N + D)\ (\pm M)$ may help to increase that possibility.

It would be well to conclude here with a statement by Dr. Ernest Dichter [7], "Possessions are tangible expressions of our attitude towards life. It is important to understand what objects mean to us before we can market them or communicate about them."

Appearance–Embroidery, Candor or Confusion

What we generally hope will be transmitted by product appearance is a veracious and desirable message. If that message expresses a promise which the product is seen to fulfill, then it becomes the stimulus for action–usually in the form of acquisition, specification, or purchase. This holds true whether we are dealing with typewriters or tractors. Where appearance communication is garbled, unconvincing, deceptive, or lacks clarity, then the product will be passively ignored or actively rejected. "I wouldn't own it if they gave it to me," is an example of failure of communication. This can also happen if the visual information is inappropriate or inconsistent with the user's previous expectations. A few examples follow.

The most obvious information coding is color. Bananas are generally accepted when yellow, ignored when green, and rejected if black. Another example would be if the familiar "Coke" bottle were used to merchandise milk—picture the suspicious white substance which would be displayed; it is likely that this inappropriate message would create confusion and perhaps revulsion. In this case, shape and contour as appearance factors conflict with color. Similar effects can be experienced if we exchange the color and textural characteristics between watermelon and bread. White watermelons and red bread are likely to create responses that are not apt to be positive. Such conditions, however, are mainly examples of error, not fabrication.

Deliberate transfer of configuration style has also been made in products wherein stoves come to resemble computers and electric fans resemble jet engines. At times, such myths are successfully accepted when associative or social values bestow superior attributes to them. When appearance is borrowed in this way, it is often accepted if it has a popularized meaning within the specific market. This is not to condone styling that is imitative or gimmicky but merely explains why superficial designs are perpetrated. George Nelson, one of the foremost U. S. designers, humorously puts down this practice [*8*],

> We live in a dynamic period. Movement is one of the things that tends to stimulate and excite us and the product has to move. If it moves at a slow rate, something must be done to the styling to, at the least, increase the visual miles per hour. And, it is characteristic of the successful small consumer product that it says very clearly that it is going somewhere with a purpose, with a great thrust in a hurry.

Like other forms of communication, appearance can be truthful or imaginative and this depends on the motivation of its user. Pretense, however, must be understood for what it is. It can have disastrous market results. The legend of the Edsel is a case in point; it communicated gaudiness and epitomized conspicuous consumption, gross affluence, and many of the values from which the public was then turning away. This attitude, in fact, foreshadowed market interest in the compact car and the sports car. No question that an appearance message was communicated albeit, not the one intended. The clear response was "we don't want any."

Inappropriate use of materials can cause the same effect. Recently, an attempt to use the waxed-type milk container as a consumer package for non-edible substances such as toiletries, medicinals, and garden chemicals was tried. These packages failed and were forced off the market. The wax container was too well associated with comestibles, besides which its inadvertant use by children was hazardous. Functionally, it was probably an excellent container, however, the appearance statement as conveyed by choice of material was wrong. Communication, in the examples stated, was dependent on visual signals inherent in appearance of the material itself and in its associated values.

The choice of what products are to say is an ethical one. Some products tolerate little license because neither function, tradition, nor historical usage will permit mendacity. Musical instruments, hand tools, and sports equipment are good examples. There are products, however, which are not so restricted and in which veracity is bent 90 deg. Packaging which holds less than it offers, toys that prove fragile and frustrating, appliances that sprout more controls than convenience, furniture which is marginal but "looks like a million"—are all testimony to cost pressures which result in accepted hanky-panky. Design is often caught in the middle as the courier. Appearance factors in themselves, no more than language, are devoid of ethical values but their use in design is not. The objective of industry is to sell goods, which is often linked to something called "eye-appeal." The dichotomy for both the designer and manufacturer is in determining reasonable limits between minimum competitive attention and visual forgery. For many, the guidelines are still in dispute. For some, misrepresentation is a way of life. For others, an occasional counterfeit is permissable. For all, reputation is at stake while both consumer and government wait to detect any contradiction between message and performance.

The person who instruments these implications for better or worse, is the designer and it is upon him that the burden falls heaviest—for it is he who becomes the lonely custodian of communication. Embroidery or candor is a question always in the balance; professional design has always struggled for the latter, but it is primarily society which will determine the choice.

Significance of Product Communication

Our technological society has forced us into a greater dialogue with the object. Whether we operate a toaster or a space capsule, whether we are purchasers or specifiers, observers or operators, we are dependent upon information, which must be accurate, meaningful, and fast. This applies even to such whimsical and presumably unessential artifacts as toys which can possess the ability to guide safe behavior and express play value. Can we accept less from more serious goods? The need is for more penetrating application of appearance factors which has daily and unavoidable significance for millions of people.

I am inclined to believe that such abused words as "good taste" or "good design" have less to do with aesthetic or esoteric considerations than with satisfying communication. Good design is good communication, and good communication is successful design. Whether it be a consumer, scientific, or industrial product, appearance establishes the first rapport with the prospective user. It identifies the function of the object and reflects the symbolic and humanistic attributes needed to evoke an empathic response. Appearance must communicate these relationships in instantaneous, non-verbal ways. In bottom-line terms, it must command attention, bespeak believability, support price, and project the reputation of the maker.

In new and innovative products, it is even more essential that communication be understood for it must express ideas which have no precedent. This requires sophistication in appearance syntax; if communication is ambiguous, the product is a step closer to failure.

A method of appearance interpretation and analysis is overdue, and the threshold of such a technique lies ahead. The applications are wide and easily stated. We require the ability to know what we are saying. We must communicate a product's compatability to its function and its environment. We must satisfy the user's needs and aspirations in a visually self-evident way. We must convey intrinsic appeal in terms of useful social and personal values. We must transmit information and provide redeemable expectations. We must be able to test the rightness of a design by what it communicates. Finally, we depend upon appearance components as a media to explain technology.

When product appearance is successful, it is because it communicates a visually articulated need. Among other things, the design will state that it performs, that it serves a purpose, that it conveys reliability, and, that it reinforces the choice of the user. Altogether, it is a badge of the company's marketing personality expressed in one object—it reveals the craftsmanship and value being held out. Product appearance broadcasts such evidence continuously. Its non-verbal address enhances the desire to use and possess for its intrinsic qualities. Where these conditions are met, product appearance serves industry's objectives, as well as its customers.

Understanding appearance values may lead us to techniques for better product communication. This would be valuable not only to the designer's understanding, but also in better fulfilling user requirements. Such techniques would also be of import to management which seeks quantifiable answers in areas in which it is about to make substantial dollar commitments.

Product appearance now emerges from the experience and intuitive creativity of the form giver. Some employ a methodology. The design personality develops and expresses Communication Value (*Cv*) in a way in which others are not trained to do. This capability also depends upon sensitivity to materials, to people, to aesthetics, and to associative meanings. The validity of the designers approach is only confirmed by market response. Satisfying complex and often conflicting product requirements could be made more manageable as we approach a science of appearance factors.

Conclusion

In conclusion, it would be well to consider a point expressed in a statement by Art Kane [*9*], a well-known contemporary photographer and artist.

> A man who communicates through a machine must supersede the machine, must overpower it. Machines are tolerable only when they respond to man's desires and impulses, only when they are the slaves and we are the masters—they otherwise breed repetition, monotony and destruction.

References

[*1*] Hunter, R. S. in *Appearance of Metallic Surfaces, ASTM STP 478*, American Society for Testing and Materials, 1970, pp. 3-21.

[*2*] Gombrich, E. H., "The Visual Image," *Scientific American*, Sept. 1972.

[*3*] Latham, R. S., *Who Designs America?* L. B. Holland, Ed., Anchor Books, Doubleday & Co., New York, 1966, pp. 257-280.

[*4*] Mussen, P. H., Conger, J. J., and Kagan, J., *Child Development and Personality*, 3rd ed, Harper & Row, New York, 1963, pp. 157-170.

[*5*] Olds, James, "Pleasure Centers in the Brain—Frontiers of Psychological Research Readings from *Scientific American*," *Scientific American*, Oct. 1956.

[*6*] Ruesch, Jargen, and Kees, Weldon, *Non-Verbal Communication—Notes on the Visual Perception of Human Relations*, University of California Press, Berkeley, Calif., 1964, pp. 6-8, 12, 27, 90, 96, 100, 190-191.

[*7*] Dichter, Ernest, "The Psychology of the World of Objects," *Handbook of Consumer Motivations*, McGraw-Hill, New York, 1964.

[*8*] Nelson, George in *Communication—The Art of Understanding and Being Understood*, Hastings House, New York, 1963, p. 63.

[*9*] Kane, Art in *Communication—The Art of Understanding and Being Understood*, Hastings House, New York, 1963, p. 63.

Bibliography

Foster, Dean and Danker, W. H. in *Basic Principles of Sensory Evaluation, ASTM STP 433*, American Society for Testing and Materials, 1968, pp. 7-10.

Sherrington, C. S., *Integrative Action of the Nervous System*, Yale University Press, New Haven, Conn., 1920.

Stone, Herbert and Pangborn, R. M. in *Basic Principles of Sensory Evaluation, ASTM STP 433*, American Society for Testing and Materials, 1968, pp. 30-46.

Klemmer, E. T. in *Basic Principles of Sensory Evaluation, ASTM STP 433*, American Society for Testing and Materials, 1968, pp. 51-57.

Perin, Constance, *With Man in Mind—An Interdisciplinary Prospectus for Environmental Design*, MIT Press, Cambridge, Mass., 1970, pp. 15, 39.

C. A. Burnham[1] *and C. T. Grimm*[1]

Connotative Meaning of Visual Properties of Surfaces

REFERENCE: Burnham, C. A. and Grimm, C. T., "**Connotative Meaning of Visual Properties of Surfaces,**" *Sensory Evaluation of Appearance of Materials, ASTM STP 545,* American Society for Testing and Materials, 1973, pp. 54-69.

ABSTRACT: The goals of the research efforts described in this paper were (1) to establish a rational technique for the selection of the visual properties of architectural surfaces and (2) to determine the psychophysical relationships between objective measurements of surfaces and their psychological meaning. Respondents rated samples of architectural surfaces (brick surfaces varying in size, texture, and color) and design concepts (home, prison, etc.) on a series of bipolar adjective scales selected to measure the meaning of the object on the three commonly identified dimensions of connotative meaning–the evaluative, potency, and activity dimensions (the semantic differential technique). The validity and reliability of this application of the semantic differential were assessed and found to be satisfactory.

Since each rated object receives a score on each of the three dimensions and can be localized as a point in three-dimensional semantic space, one can obtain quantitative differences between the connotative meaning of diverse objects. A rational technique for the selection of the visual properties of architectural surfaces would involve selecting surfaces whose meaning matched the meaning of the design concept.

Psychophysical relationships were obtained between the meaning of the visual properties of the surfaces on each of the dimensions of connotative meaning and physical measurements of the surfaces. Several of these relationships indicated an association between the physical and psychological aspects of the surfaces. Hence, it is probable that surfaces could be manufactured which would permit one to obtain a close match between the meaning of the surfaces and the meaning of design concepts.

The results of these preliminary studies indicate that further research on the connotative meaning of visual properties of surfaces is warranted.

KEY WORDS: senses, perception, visual perception, psychological effects, surfaces

The design criteria which govern an architect's choice of building materials are primarily engineering, economics, and aesthetics. There has been a

[1] Associate professor, Psychology, and associate director, Center for Building Research, respectively, University of Texas, Austin, Tex. 78712.

considerable amount of research on the engineering and economic aspects of building materials. Thus, there is a rational basis for decision on these two criteria. There is, however, no rational basis for aesthetic decisions. Architects select surface materials which they feel best express the design concept of the building they are designing. An architect's judgment of the best or most aesthetically pleasing surface is based on informed intuition and rather vague principles of good design. The aesthetic criteria cannot be stated explicitly in the way that the engineering and economic criteria can. There are no formulae for the aesthetic decision. In this paper we propose a method for the selection of the visual properties of architectural surfaces.

The method follows from a particular set of considerations or premises. It should be realized from the onset that our method is only one of a number of possible methods that could be generated. Furthermore, we do not anticipate or wish that it be followed slavishly. The method is developed in the context of the appropriate choice of surface properties of brick for building types. The method can, however, be applied to the selection of any surface appearance for any purpose. The selection method also produces a rationale for obtaining psychophysical relationships between objective measurements of surfaces and the psychological response to the appearance of the surfaces in order to understand the basis for the psychological response to the appearance of a surface.

Our psychological approach to the selection of the visual properties of architectural surfaces evolved from the following considerations. An architect has a design concept which he attempts to express in the building's spatial form and specific visual properties of the material surfaces, such as color, texture, shape, size, and pattern. The building expresses the meaning of the design concept. Thus, the idea of a prison as a social rehabilitation center is expressed by visual properties of surfaces which would be quite different than those used to express the idea of a prison as a place for punishment. Depending on the idea of the design concept, textures can be course or fine, colors gray or bright, illumination dull or light, space closed or open, distances great or intimate, and patterns regular or variegated. The architect presumably attempts to match the meaning of the design concept with the building form and the visual properties of the surface materials. Our selection technique involves measuring the meaning of the design concept and the meaning of visual properties of architectural surfaces, and then selecting a surface whose visual properties most nearly match the meaning of the design concept. The semantic differential is used to measure the connotative meaning of the design concept and the surfaces.

Semantic Differential Methodology

Objects have two types of meaning, denotative meaning (what the object is) and connotative meaning (one's emotional response to the object). "Home" denotes, according to the dictionary, a family's place of residence. "Home" connotes, according to our respondents, something that is pleasant rather than unpleasant, soft rather than hard, and relaxed rather than tense. Clearly, the connotative meanings of buildings and materials are to be matched if the building is to be expressive of a design concept. One would hardly use materials that are thought of as delicate, soft, yielding, or weak to express a design concept which is high in potency.

Dr. Charles Osgood, a psychologist at the University of Illinois, has developed a test instrument, termed the semantic differential, to measure the connotative meaning of objects [*1*].[2] Respondents are asked to rate objects against a series of seven-point scales labeled at the ends by polar adjectives such as pleasant-unpleasant, soft-hard, and relaxed-tense. Osgood and his associates had many different people rate many different concepts or objects against a large number of such polar adjective scales. These ratings were factor analyzed to determine the dimensions along which the connotative meanings of objects vary. They found that three independent dimensions account for more than 75 percent of the variance of the connotative meaning of objects or concepts. These dimensions and examples of polar adjective pairs used to measure them are:

Evaluation dimension
- beautiful-ugly
- pleasant-unpleasant
- harmonious-dissonant
- meaningful-meaningless
- cheerful-sad
- refined-vulgar

Potency dimension
- rugged-delicate
- hard-soft
- tenacious-yielding
- strong-weak
- tough-tender
- masculine-feminine

Activity dimension
- energetic-inert
- tense-relaxed
- dynamic-static
- interesting-boring
- warm-cold
- fast-slow

Several other investigators have applied the semantic differential to architectural problems. The primary concern of such research has been to determine

[2] The italic numbers in brackets refer to the list of references appended to this paper.

the dimensions along which buildings or architectural spaces vary. Unfortunately, the output of factor analysis—the statistical technique used to determine the dimensions—depends to a great extent upon the input. The words chosen for the ratings and the nature of the buildings or spaces which are rated will influence the obtained dimensions of meaning. Since we are attempting to compare two quite different sorts of concepts, building types and visual properties of architectural surfaces, we elected to use the dimensions obtained by Osgood and his colleagues. However, other polar-adjective pairs and other combinations of the adjectives for the dimensions might be more appropriate for specific building types, as is indicated by Collins' study of libraries [*2*], or for certain aspects of architectural spaces, as is suggested by Canter's report [*3*].

To obtain the connotative meaning of an object or concept, one asks a respondent to indicate on a seven-point scale between each polar adjective pair the point which best describes the relationship or association between the concept and the adjectives. A check mark at the ends of the scales, next to one of the adjectives, indicates that the concept is very closely related to the adjective. A check mark at the midpoint of the scale indicates either that the concept is equally associated with both adjectives, or that the adjectives are unrelated in any way to the concept. Each scale position is assigned a number from +3 to −3. (Conventionally, the evaluative, potent, and active ends of the scales are assigned the positive number.) The connotative meaning of an object on each dimension is taken as the mean of the ratings given the concept by all respondents on all polar adjective scales used to measure the dimension.

The space defined by the possible loci of a concept on the three dimensions, arranged orthogonally in Cartesian coordinates, is referred to as semantic space. Any given concept has one position in this space. The distance between the meanings of two concepts, such as a design concept and a visual surface property, is easily calculated by applying the formula

$$D_{ds} = [(E_d - E_s)^2 + (P_d - P_s)^2 + (A_d - A_s)^2]^{0.5}$$

where

D_{ds} = distance between the meaning of a design concept and a visual property of a surface in semantic spatial units,
E = evaluative coordinate,
P = potency coordinate,
A = activity coordinate,
d = subscript indicative of the design concept, and
s = subscript indicative of the visual property of the surface.

In principle then, the technique of measuring the connotative meaning of a design concept and various visual properties of surfaces offers a rational basis for the selection of a particular surface. One simply selects that particular surface which matches the design concept, that is, the most similar in connotative meaning to the concept. Mathematically, one attempts to minimize D_{ds}.

The information that a surface material with certain visual properties is located at a particular position in semantic space is all that is necessary for the employment of this selection technique. It would, however, be interesting and useful to discover the specific physical attributes of surface material which are associated with the psychological response to that material as measured by the semantic differential. If variation of a specifiable physical dimension were correlated with variation of some aspect of the psychological response to that material, one could attempt to design novel surfaces which would be expected to produce a predicted psychological response. A surface could be designed to fill in a gap in semantic space, or a surface could be designed to maximize the psychological response on one or more of the three dimensions of connotative meaning. Obtaining such psychophysical relationships would also serve to link the physical properties of the surfaces with their psychological effects.

Several investigations were conducted with students of architecture, architectural engineering, and psychology in which the semantic differential technique was used to measure the connotative meaning of the visual properties of brick textures, colors, and sizes and shapes. The obtained semantic space coordinates for various brick surface properties are reported. These ratings may be useful to designers interested in applying the proposed rational selection precedure. However, the representativeness of these data should be checked against data collected from different samples before they are used for this purpose. We used these ratings to assess the reliability and validity of the semantic differential technique as applied to visual properties of surfaces, to assess the proposed selection technique, and to obtain certain psychophysical relationships.

Semantic Differential Ratings

Texture

Forty-two undergraduate students from an introductory psychology course viewed ten colored slides of 2 by 4 ft (61 by 122 cm) panels of standard modular brick laid in running bond. Five textures were studied. Each texture was presented in a dark color (ISCC-NBS, No. 19, grayish-red) and a light color (ISCC-NBS No. 73, pale orange-yellow). Each panel was rated on 12 semantic differential scales, four scales for each of the three dimensions of semantic space. The average rating for each texture on these dimensions is shown in Table 1. Positive numbers are good, strong, and active on a +3 to −3 scale in this and the other tables. A statistical analysis of these data showed that the textures differ significantly on each of the three dimensions of connotative meaning. In general, brick textures are neither good nor bad, but they may be strong or weak, active or passive. All textures in dark brick were considered strong, the dark scratch

TABLE 1–*Semantic space coordinates for five brick textures of two lightnesses.*

Dimension	Lightness	Texture					
		Average	Rock	Scratch	Dent	Velour	Uneven
E_S	Light	0.22	0.76	−0.34	0.31	0.30	0.07
Evaluative	Dark	0.27	0.49	0.31	0.60	0.02	−0.07
(Good-Bad)	Average	0.25	0.63	−0.02	0.45	0.16	0.0
P_S	Light	−0.01	−0.03	0.51	−0.18	0.33	−0.68
Potency	Dark	1.19	1.15	1.71	0.82	1.43	0.85
(Strong-Weak)	Average	0.59	0.56	1.11	0.32	0.88	0.08
A_S	Light	−0.35	0.12	−0.38	0.52	−0.77	−1.22
Activity	Dark	0.19	0.36	0.22	1.29	−0.20	−0.70
(Active-Passive)	Average	−0.08	0.24	−0.08	0.90	−0.48	−0.96

being the strongest. The light uneven texture is the weakest. Dark dent texture is active, and light brick in uneven and velour texture are passive.

These students also rated ten building types on the same semantic differential scales and made direct suitability judgments of brick texture-color combinations for the building types. These data were used to assess the validity of the semantic differential ratings and the proposed selection criterion.

Color

Twelve sheets of colored paper, 9 by 11 in. (229 by 279 mm), representing specific brick colors were rated on 18 semantic differential scales by 35 architecture students. The mean ratings on each of six scales were averaged to obtain a rating for each of the three semantic dimensions. The coordinates in semantic space of each color are given in Table 2. From these data, few unglazed brick colors are either good or bad. Many unglazed brick colors are either active or passive. Moderate orange is the most active, and brownish pink is the most passive. Many brick colors are either strong or weak. Of those colors tested, grayish reddish brown is the strongest, and pale yellowish pink is the weakest.

These architectural students rerated four of these colored sheets one month later. The rerating data were used to assess the reliability of the semantic differential ratings.

Size and Shape

Black and white photographic projection slides of brick panels constructed from brick of four different sizes were rated by 21 architectural engineering students and 36 students from an introductory psychology course. The four brick sizes studied were: economy norman, economy, standard, and Roman.

TABLE 2–*Coordinates in semantic space for twelve unglazed brick colors.*

Color	Munsell No.	ISCC-NBS No.	Evaluative (Good-Bad) E_S	Potency (Strong-Weak) P_S	Activity (Active-Passive) A_S
Grayish red	4.0 R 4.4/4.8	19	–0.28	1.08	0.31
Pale yellowish pink	4.2 YR 8.6/2.2	31	0.44	–1.49	–0.87
Brownish pink	7.0 YR 7.1/2.3	33	–0.51	–0.53	–0.99
Grayish reddish brown	9.0 R 3.4/2.4	46	–0.77	1.36	–0.16
Moderate orange	4.6 YR 6.5/8.2	53	0.15	1.00	1.69
Light brown	5.4 YR 5.4/4.8	57	–0.81	0.77	–0.11
Light grayish brown	6.4 YR 5.4/2.2	60	–1.12	0.54	–0.84
Grayish brown	5.5 YR 3.5/1.8	61	–0.44	1.19	–0.21
Light yellowish brown	8.7 YR 6.5/5.0	76	0.77	–0.32	0.58
Pale yellow	4.7 Y 9.0/3.8	89	0.82	–1.15	–0.42
Dark grayish yellow	3.8 Y 5.9/9.0	91	0.14	0.84	–0.44
Grayish yellow	3.8 Y 7.4/1.4	93	0.65	–0.79	–0.17

Two 2 by 4 ft (61 by 122 cm) panels were made with each brick size. One was horizontally oriented (2 ft high by 4 ft wide) and the other vertically oriented (4 ft high by 2 ft wide). The brick were laid in a running bond pattern. Ratings were made on 18 semantic differential scales, six for each dimension. Table 3 presents the average ratings for these four brick sizes. The data are averaged over the two groups of students and over the horizontal and vertical panels, since these variables produced little difference in the position of a brick size on a dimension of semantic space. The potency ratings of these four sizes vary considerably, the evaluative ratings vary somewhat less, and the activity ratings are all close to the midpoint of the dimension. These size ratings were used to relate dimensional measurements of brick to the dimensions of connotative meaning. These same students also made a judgment of the aesthetic pleasantness of each of the eight panels. These ratings are discussed in conjunction with the validity of the semantic differential.

Reliability of the Ratings

The reliability of a test instrument is indicated by the consistency of measurements obtained with it. There are two types of test reliability, intra-subject reliability and inter-subject reliability. The intra-subject reliability of semantic differential ratings of visual surfaces was assessed by comparing the ratings of the colored sheets made by architectural students approximately one month apart. Twelve colors were rated on the first administration and a selected group of four colors, representing a range of lightness from yellow to brown, were rerated during the second administration. The average absolute mean difference, averaged across the three dimensions of connotative meaning and the four colors, between the two sets of ratings was 0.28 semantic scale units. This represents relatively small changes from one administration to the next. This figure can be compared with the average range of these four colors on the three dimensions of connotative meaning which was 1.85 semantic scale units.

The question of inter-subject reliability was assessed by comparing the ratings of brick sizes made by architectural engineering students with the ratings made by students from an introductory psychology course. These two groups of students are quite different. The architectural engineering students are under-

TABLE 3–*Semantic space coordinates for four brick sizes.*

Unit	Nominal Face Areas, in.^{2}	Nominal Length, in.	Nominal Height, in.	Ratio of Length to Height	Semantic Dimension E_s	P_s	A_s
Roman	24	12	2	6	−0.32	−0.64	−0.12
Standard Modular	21.4	8	2.67	3	0.74	0.08	0.28
Economy Norman	48	12	4	3	0.74	1.14	−0.34
Economy	32	8	4	2	−0.24	0.55	−0.25

going professional training and are likely to become designers. The introductory psychology students are quite representative of liberal arts students and are likely to become consumers of architectural products. The average absolute mean difference, averaged across the three dimensions of connotative meaning and the four brick sizes studied, was 0.23 semantic scale units. This figure indicates that these brick were rated in a similar manner by the two groups. In summation, the semantic differential provides reliable measurements of visual surfaces, although, as is true for all psychological tests, care must be taken to ensure cooperative and well-motivated respondents to obtain reliable data.

Validity of the Ratings

To be useful, a measurement technique must be valid; it must measure what it purports to measure. The validity of the semantic differential is difficult to assess, because there are no other instruments to measure connotative meaning. The semantic differential has been widely used in psychological research, and it is a highly regarded test instrument [*4*].

One way to consider the validity of semantic differential ratings is to compare the ratings of familiar objects on the semantic differential dimensions with one's intuitive impression of these objects. This allows one to estimate the apparent or face validity of the semantic differential. The introductory psychology students who rated the brick textures also rated ten building types on the same semantic differential scales. These data are shown in Table 4. Consider the relative ratings of the two building types "prison" and "home." Prison was rated very low on the evaluative dimension, whereas home was rated very high. Prison was not very active, whereas home was somewhat active. These ratings correspond to common

TABLE 4—*Semantic space coordinates for ten building types.*

	Dimension		
Building Type	Evaluative (Good-Bad) E_d	Potency (Strong-Weak) P_d	Activity (Active-Passive) A_d
Courthouse	0.90	1.62	0.54
Elementary School	0.88	0.18	0.16
Home	2.19	−0.46	0.79
Hospital	0.98	0.22	0.40
Hotel	1.55	0.20	0.93
Industrial Research Laboratory	0.71	1.39	0.85
Office Building	1.26	0.82	0.90
Prison	−1.08	2.13	−0.24
Shopping Center	1.21	0.37	0.82
Warehouse	−1.05	1.77	−1.01
Average	0.76	0.82	0.41

sense impressions of home and prison and thus support the validity of the semantic differential.

In the study of brick sizes, the architectural engineering and introductory psychology students who rated the eight panels on the semantic differential scales also rated them on a seven-point scale of aesthetic pleasantness, running from not pleasant to very pleasant. The economy norman and the standard modular brick face sizes were judged as being most aesthetically pleasant and were also highest on the evaluative dimension of the semantic differential (see Table 3). The economy and the Roman brick face sizes were judged as least pleasant and were lowest on the evaluative dimension. This finding of a relationship between the evaluative dimension and a general rating of aesthetic pleasantness corresponds to common sense impressions and thus, like the building type ratings, helps to confirm the validity of semantic differential ratings of the visual properties of architectural surfaces. The fact that there was no correlation between the aesthetic pleasantness ratings and the other dimensions of connotative meaning is important, because it shows that the position in semantic space of a visual property of a brick surface depends on more than a global impression of its aesthetic pleasantness.

Validity of the Selection Technique

The validity of using the semantic differential to relate design concepts and visual properties of architectural surfaces was investigated by comparing selections made from semantic differential judgments with direct judgments of suitability. A ten by ten matrix of the distance in semantic space between each building type and each brick texture-shade combination was calculated from the ratings of the introductory psychology students. (The texture-shade ratings are shown in Table 1; the building type ratings in Table 4. The distances were calculated by applying the distance formula to each of the 100 texture-shade, building type pairings.) The texture-shade closest in meaning to the meaning of the building type "home" was light-rock; the brick furthest from "home" was dark-velour. The dark-velour brick were located in semantic space near the courthouse, prison, and warehouse building types.

During the same testing session these students made direct judgments of the suitability of each of the ten texture-shade combinations for the building types. They were reshown the slides of the ten brick panels and asked to state the three building types they thought the particular texture-shade combination was most suitable for. A ten by ten matrix of suitability judgments was calculated from these responses. There was a moderate, although not perfect, correlation between the matrix of direct suitability judgments and the matrix of semantic space distances. The light-rock brick was judged as most suitable for a home. The dark-velour brick was among the brick judged as least suitable for a home, and it was one of the brick judged as most suitable for a courthouse, prison, and warehouse.

The fact that there was a moderate agreement between the two matrices indicates that the semantic differential technique for selecting an architectural surface is not completely out of line with other more direct techniques. If, however, there was perfect agreement between the two techniques, there would be no reason to use the semantic differential, which is the more tedious to apply. It is probable that the distances in semantic space more closely reflect the fit between the design concept and the visual properties of the surface, since semantic differential ratings, unlike direct suitability judgments, minimize the influence of exposure to texture-shade, building type pairings in the environment.

Psychophysical Relationships

To understand the basis for the obtained semantic differential ratings of the visual properties of brick surfaces, we obtained physical measurements of texture, size and shape, and color to correlate with the obtained semantic differential ratings. These psychophysical relationships result in a better understanding of the basis for variations in the connotative meaning of visual properties of surface.

Texture

Physical roughness characteristics of six brick textures were measured by the technique of microtopography, using an instrument developed by Dr. Clyde Lee. This instrument consists of a needle point which is passed over the textured surface and measures the surface profile at 0.0033 in. (0.0838 mm) intervals horizontally and 0.000042 in. (0.00107 mm) intervals vertically. The readings of the needle can be displayed as a texture profile of the surface. The texture can be quantified by computing variables such as height of peaks, depth of valleys, density of peaks, variances of slopes, etc. We looked at the relationship between a number of these physical measurements of texture and the semantic differential ratings of the textures. The only association between these roughness measurements and the semantic differential ratings was an association between the number of positive peaks having a height of 0.06 in. or more above the mean elevation of the surface and ratings on the potency dimension. As the number of positive peaks increased, the potency ratings of the brick textures first increased and then decreased. This curvilinear relationship is shown in Fig. 1.

The technique of microtopography is only one of several ways of measuring surface roughness. This technique and the specific measures of roughness were devised to predict friction of road surfaces. Other techniques or other measures of roughness might produce more associations with measures of connotative meaning.

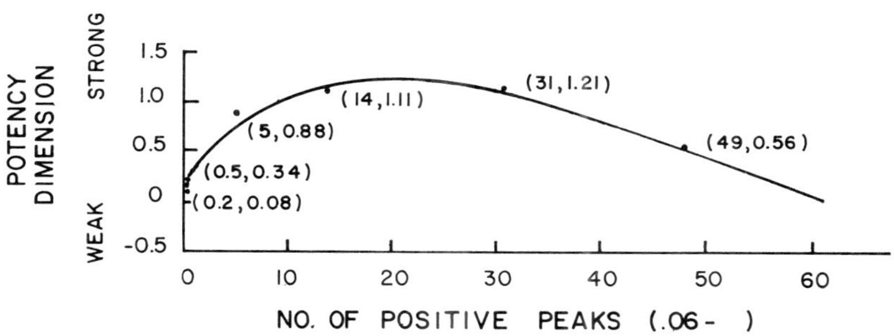

FIG. 1—*Psychophysical relationship between texture and connotative meaning.*

Size and Shape

A similar psychophysical analysis was performed on the data from the brick size study. (The semantic differential ratings and face sizes of these brick are shown in Table 3, the psychophysical relationships are shown in Fig. 2.) It is possible to relate a particular physical property of these brick to their ordering on each of the three dimensions of connotative meaning. The physical property related to the evaluative dimension is the length to height ratio. The two brick with a length to height ratio of 3, the economy norman and standard modular brick, received the highest ratings on this dimension. The evaluative ratings decreased as the ratio deviated from this value. The physical dimension most closely associated with the potency dimension is the height of the brick. For these brick, laid in running bond, the potency ratings decline as the brick height decreases. The ratings on the activity dimension reflect the area of the brick. The brick with the smallest face area is the most active. As the area increases, the activity ratings decrease. These relationships need to be substantiated by additional research; they are based on only four data points. The obtained correspondences strongly suggest that brick size can be altered to achieve desired psychological effects. It is clear that it is impossible to maximize the ratings on all three dimensions with a single brick size and shape. For example, an increase in height should result in an increase in potency; but, if the length to height ratio were held at the optimum value of three, such an increase in height would also increase the face area, and thereby produce a decrease in the activity rating.

Color

The physical dimensions of color are wavelength, intensity, and purity. Alterations in these dimensions produce alterations in hue, lightness, and saturation, respectively. Are these color dimensions, as quantified by the Munsell color notation system, related to the dimensions of connotative meaning?

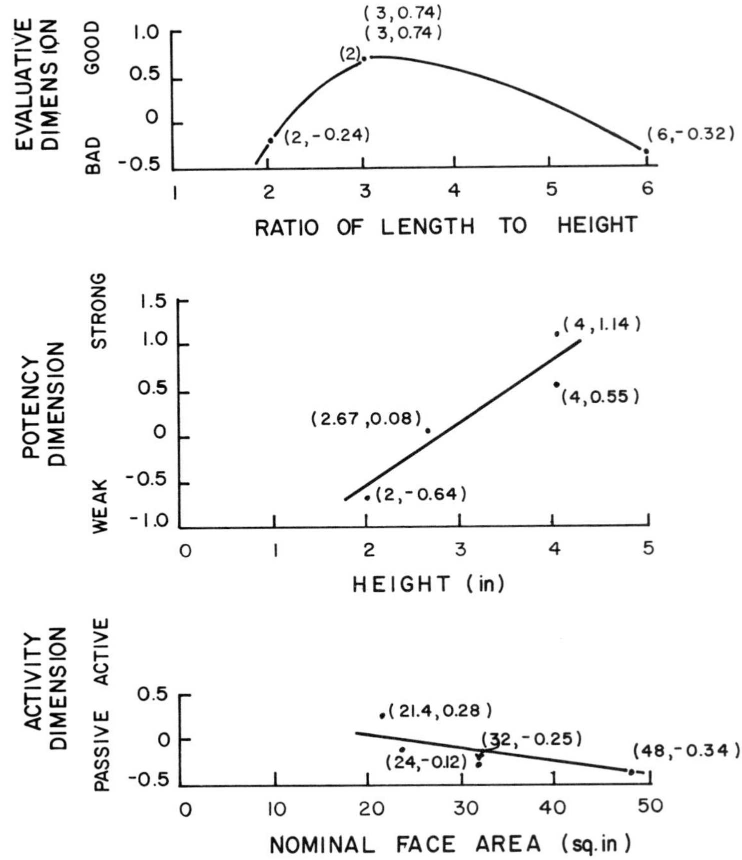

FIG. 2–*Psychophysical relationships between size and shape and connative meaning.*

Graphical plots of the relationships between the Munsell hue, value (lightness), and chroma (saturation) of the 12 colored sheets rated by the architectural students and the ratings on the three dimensions of connotative meaning are shown in Fig. 3. (The semantic differential ratings of these colors are shown in Table 2.) These data suggest that as hue changes from red to yellow, the ratings on the evaluative dimension increase and the potency ratings decrease. The same relationships hold for value (lightness). As lightness increases, evaluative ratings increase and potency ratings decrease. An increase in chroma (saturation) produces an increase in activity. The actual psychophysical relationships for color may be cleaner than those indicated in the graphs of Fig. 3, since the rated papers varied on more than one dimension. Thus, the large scatter from the line

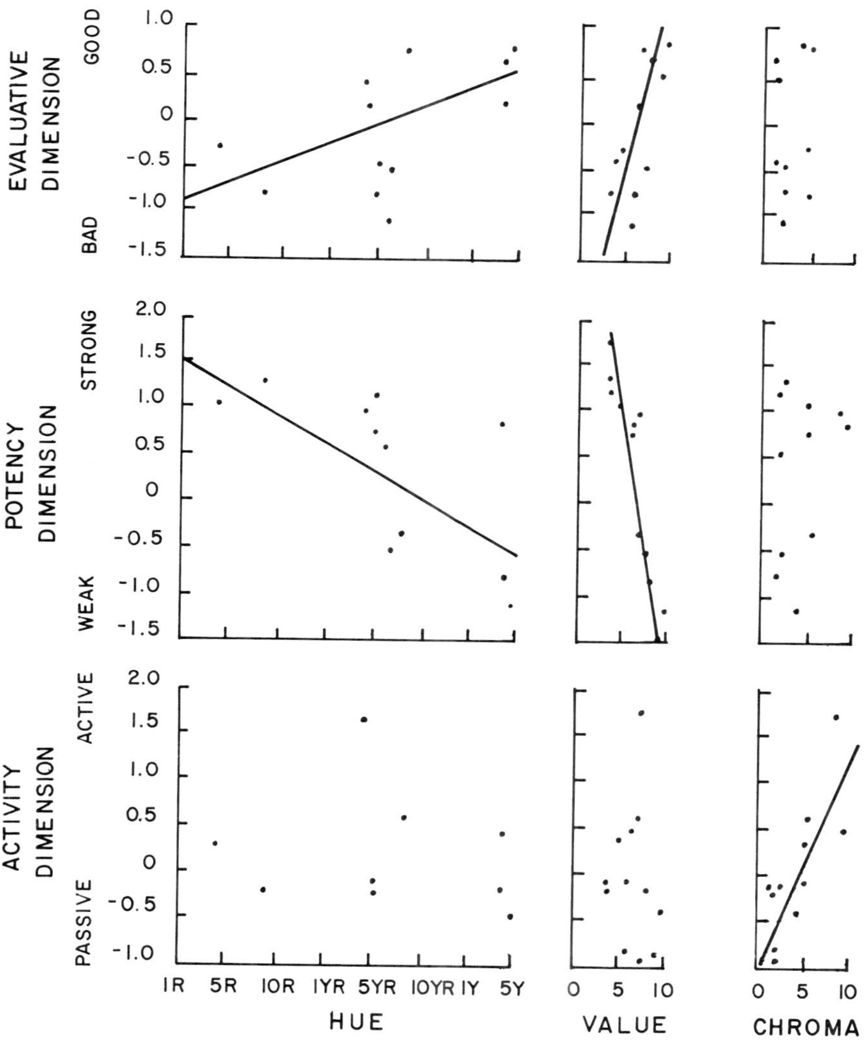

FIG. 3–*Psychophysical relationships between color and connotative meaning.*

relating hue and the evaluative dimension may be attributed to psychological differences produced by variations of value and chroma for approximately the same hue. It is of interest that the same linear correlations, with the possible exception of the hue-evaluative relationship, were found in an independent semantic differential color study using female college students and 16 colors spread over a wider range of the spectrum [*5*].

Discussion

The results of these investigations appear to demonstrate the viability of measuring the connotative meaning of visual properties of surfaces and using the dimensions of connotative meaning as the basis of a rational selection technique and for psychophysical relationships. However, the generality of these ratings needs to be further assessed and certain problems need to be clarified before the technique is applied. Specifically, there are issues of the applicability of the dimensions used, the generality of the panels, and the suitability of the technique for other surface properties and other materials.

The semantic differential dimensions and the polar adjectives for measuring the dimensions used in these investigations were those which previous researchers have found to be applicable to a large variety of concepts. It is possible that the connotative meaning of visual properties of surfaces might be more accurately assessed by different scales and that the dimensions of connotative meaning for surface properties are different from those found in other studies. A large-scale, factor analytic study is necessary to determine the dimensions of meaning most suitable for these applications of the semantic differential rating technique.

The panels of respondents used in these investigations were composed of students. Other populations need to be assessed to determine the generality of the particular ratings obtained in our studies. There may be systematic variations in the ratings obtained as a function of the respondents' occupation, expertise, or geographical locale. If such variations occurred, the use of the proposed selection technique and the obtained psychophysical relationships would have to be limited to a subset of the population.

These investigations were limited to measurements of the connotative meaning of brick texture, color, and size and shape. Other investigations conducted by the authors have explored the applicability of the semantic differential rating technique to other visual properties and other materials. These investigations strongly suggest that respondents can make reliable ratings of any visual property of any surface. Apparently, the semantic differential technique can be used to obtain meaningful data about the psychological response to the appearance of materials. However, more extended studies with diverse materials are definitely warranted to extend the generality of these techniques.

Finally, we do not suggest that our proposed selection procedure be employed blindly. Problems are certain to arise in its use. For example, designers would be likely to rate many design concepts near the positive end of the three dimensions of connotative meaning; unfortunately, few visual properties of surfaces are located near that position in semantic space. It might be necessary to weigh the dimensions by an importance factor to determine the most suitable surface property. And certainly other factors besides similarity in semantic space would affect the choice of a surface property for a design concept.

In summary, the theoretical considerations and experimental studies reported here represent small and tentative steps in the application of psychological techniques and methods to the measurement of the appearance of materials. We hope that these preliminary investigations will stimulate others to conduct additional studies of this selection criterion and of the relationship between physical measurements of surfaces and their psychological effects. Such studies should eventually provide a more scientific and rational basis for the design of our man-made environment.

Acknowledgments

The investigations reported in this article were supported by the Clay Products Association of the Southwest, Austin, Tex. The semantic differential ratings of the colored sheets were collected for the authors by Professor Edmund Furley, School of Architecture, University of Houston. We thank Dr. Clyde Lee, College of Engineering, University of Texas, for making it possible to use his instrument to obtain microtopography measurements of surface texture. Jim Cox, Department of Psychology, University of Texas, assisted in the analysis of these data.

References

[1] Osgood, C. E., Succi, G. J., and Tannenbau, P. H., *The Measurement of Meaning,* University of Illinois Press, Urbana, Ill., 1957.
[2] Collins, J. B., "Perceptual Dimensions of Architectural Space Validated Against Behavioral Criteria," Ph.D. thesis, University of Utah, 1969.
[3] Canter, David, *Transactions,* The Bartlett Society, Vol. VIII, 1967-1968, pp. 43-60.
[4] Snider, J. G. and Osgood, C. E., *Semantic Differential Technique,* Aldine Publishing Co., Chicago, 1969.
[5] Oyama, Tadasu, Tanaka, Yasumasa, and Chiba, Yoshio, *Japanese Psychological Research,* Vol. 4, No. 2, pp. 78-91.

M. W. Jenkins[1]

Obtaining and Summarizing Subjective Impressions for Correlation with Analytical Measurements

REFERENCE: Jenkins, M. W., **"Obtaining and Summarizing Subjective Impressions for Correlation with Analytical Measurements,"** *Sensory Evaluation of Appearance of Materials, ASTM STP 545,* American Society for Testing and Materials, 1973, pp. 70-90.

ABSTRACT: Subjective thresholds of acuity, acceptability, or preference must be obtained to assure a manufacturer that his product is desirable. Subjective tests are often costly and time consuming. This delays decision making and product improvement or availability. Therefore, much effort has been extended in recent years to relate subjective impressions to analytical measurements such that a subjective study need not be run each time a product is tested.

The intent of this paper is to present a few studies, initiated to evaluate product appearance, wherein statistical techniques have been interrelated to obtain and describe the relationship between subjective impressions and objective measurements. The techniques used to obtain and summarize subjective impressions are presented in some detail. They are not necessarily new and are not all-inclusive but are applicable for testing a variety of products with modifications dictated by the product tested or the threshold level of subjects. The emphasis in experimental design is on the scaling of items by rank order or paired comparison techniques.

KEY WORDS: senses, perception, consumers, product development, quality control, statistical techniques

Subjective evaluation has been defined as the process of using people to obtain measurements. Manufacturers try to provide the consumer with the product that he wants—new products, products improved aesthetically, more durable products, and products more convenient to maintain. Subjective impressions must frequently be recorded and summarized to evaluate and compare products since analytical devices are not available to assess the

[1] Statistician, Applied Statistics Section, Engineering Department, E. I. du Pont de Nemours & Co., Wilmington, Del. 19898.

acceptability or desirability of the total product, or even many of its components. It is difficult or perhaps impossible, for example, to analytically record the taste of a beverage, the drape of a fabric, the smell of a paint, or the overall appearance of a product. Even with properties that can be measured analytically such as fabric elasticity, dye uniformity, and whiteness retention, subjective thresholds of acuity, acceptability, or preference must be obtained to assure that the product is desirable. A manufacturer cannot afford to allocate research money to the development of a product of marginal appeal or to the tightening of quality control limits when the improvements in quality cannot be observed.

Subjective data are often costly and take longer to collect than analytical data, delaying decision making and, therefore, product improvement or availability. Considerable care must be used in designing and running subjective tests to assure reliable and representative data. Therefore, much effort has been extended in recent years to relate subjective impressions to analytical measurements such that a subjective study does not have to be run each time a product is tested.

The intent of this paper is to present a few studies wherein statistical techniques have been interrelated to obtain and describe the relationship between subjective impressions and objective measurements. The techniques used to obtain and summarize subjective impressions are presented in some detail. They are not neccessarily new and are not all-inclusive but are applicable for testing a variety of products with modifications dictated by the product tested or the threshold level of subjects. The emphasis in experimental design is on the scaling of items by rank order or paired comparison techniques. The studies that I have chosen were initiated to evaluate product appearance. Fiber, fabric, and garment manufacturers test their products for appearance for a variety of reasons. Not only are desirable levels of sheen, lustre, and texture important in a fabric, but the fabric must have a uniform appearance and be able to retain that appearance.

Classes of Problems

There are three major areas of frequent concern where the end goal is to relate subjective responses to analytical measurements.

Fabric Aesthetics and Uniformity

Instrumentally, we can discriminate between fabrics on the basis of bulk, lustre, uniformity, etc. We have, however, two concerns: (1) do consumers agree with the analytical discrimination? and (2) what level of the property is most desirable? The level of desirability is important. We have found in studies to assess fabric softners that the softest fabrics are not necessarily the most preferred. Extremely soft fabrics feel slick to some consumers and are therefore undesirable.

Thresholds

Uniformity is another area of much concern to us. Fabric development work often includes the reduction or elimination of problems of fabric streakiness and dye matching. Ideally, quality control limits on uniformity should be set by the consumer himself. I believe that such limits benefit both the consumer and the producer. They are not arbitrarily stringent, creating an economic problem for the manufacturer. The consumer benefits by receiving a desirable product at a lower cost. We attempt to achieve this goal and retain an efficient evaluation system by relating subjective perceptions of uniformity to analytical measurements of uniformity. The remaining step is to find that analytical value which corresponds to the subjective threshold; that is, the point above which nonuniformities are observable or objectionable.

Overall Preferences

The prediction of overall preference is always of prime concern. This, however, is extremely difficult. Opinions change with the type and amount of advertising used, the price, the introduction of competitive products, an increase in the consumer's income, the amount of his exposure to various fibers, etc. Perhaps, the most that we can expect to do is to find the key factors that explain overall preference at the time. Often these factors are also subjective and are not themselves easily correlated to objective data. If the objective of a study is to find the most preferred item of several candidate items or to see if a new product is preferred to a commercial goal item, we are often satisfied with the results prior to analytical prediction. Since the purpose of this symposium is to discuss the evaluation of the appearance of products rather than the total product, my examples will fall into the first two areas; aesthetic scaling and threshold evaluation.

Assessing Subjective Impressions

Before the discussion of actual case studies, I would like to discuss the collection of subjective impressions for correlation with objective measurements in general. Let us assume that we can analytically measure the degree of fabric luster. We wish to know the relationship between analytical evaluations and subjective impressions of luster. I will briefly discuss the following items and then describe specific data collection methods in the examples.

1. The selection of items to subjectively evaluate.
2. The selection of subjects; untrained versus trained.
3. The selection of scaling techniques; ranking versus rating.

The Selection of Items

Enough items must be chosen to cover the range of the property of interest, such as fabric luster from low to high. Frequently, items that compete commercially differ only slightly in the property to be assessed. When this is the case, items must be made such that enough differences are obtained to assess the degree of correlation even though the items may not be of commercial interest. Two items that are essentially alike add nothing to describing the relationship that exists between subjective and objective data. There are, of course, cases where the objective of the experiment is to compare two items, analytically different, to see if consumers can detect the improvement or change. In this case, the selection of the items and the test procedure are different. Often, commercial items chosen to represent acceptable levels of the property to be assessed and candidate items are included. This enables the experimenter to assess the competitability of candidates in the same experiment.

The Selection of Subjects

Trained judges or panels formed of subjects with high levels of acuity are often used for evaluations other than preference. They are familiar with the property to be evaluated, usually agree more closely with one another, and can detect smaller differences between items. The use of trained judges decreases the amount of variation in the subjective data and, thus, increases the sensitivity of the correlation relationship. If, however, the goal is to assess the reaction of the consumer as in threshold, acceptance, or preference studies, fine discrimination may not be desirable. Differences that cannot be detected by a major portion of the public present no product advantage or disadvantage. Subjects should be chosen representative of the total population associated with the product end use.

The Selection of Scaling Techniques

There are many methods and modifications of methods to subjectively scale items. Items are scaled by assigning a number to each item which represents the degree of luster associated with that item. The number can be a rating, say 1.0 to 10.0, representing no luster to maximum luster, or items can be ranked from most to least lustrous. If 10 items are ranked, a possible scale number would be 10.0 for the most lustrous item to 1.0 for the least lustrous or vice versa. Popular rating scale techniques are magnitude estimation, ratio estimation, rating by standards, and rating along an interval scale [*1,2*].[2] Ranking techniques include paired comparisons evaluating one or several pairs of items at a time to obtain a complete rank order and the ranking and rating of differences between ranks [*3*]. If one can obtain good rating data, it is always preferable. A continuum is

[2] The italic numbers in brackets refer to the list of references appended to this paper.

immediately provided and data are often normally distributed making the analysis easier and statistical tests more powerful. We have found that rating by standards using technical judges is extremely effective for wear test properties such as pill resistance and wrinkle resistance. We have not, however, been generally successful in obtaining good rating data from untrained evaluators. I usually recommend paired comparison or ranking techniques if the data are to be obtained from consumers.

Some of the problems that can occur when rating scales are used are mentioned in the following paragraph.

A person who can declare that one item is different, better than or worse than another item, will give both items the same rating if the difference is small. This is particularly true if the items are rated one at a time. Consumers use different scale lengths. Pessimists will never give an item the highest scale rating; optimists will not give the lowest. The scale length is chosen arbitrarily by the experimenter. Theoretically, the longer the scale length, the greater the ability to obtain fine discriminations. If the scale is too long, however, ratings will be bunched up at one end. If it is too short, different items obtain similar ratings. Ideally, the end points should be just below and just above the range within which a consumer can rate. Unfortunately, unless pilot studies are run, the appropriate scale length is seldom known in advance. Arithmetic adjustments can be made to put all of the data on the same scale. However, this dictates a subjective decision on the analyst's part. He must assume that subjects who rate items much alike when others do not or use only one portion of the scale, are less discriminating, or have a positive or negative bias.

Examples

The examples that follow will fall into two categories of scaling—"nominal scaling" and "ordinal scaling."

Nominal Scaling–Paired Comparisons

Occasionally we have improved a product or have changed a product in some other manner. We can detect analytical differences between the new and the old product and the only question of interest is whether the consumer will also notice this difference. Sometimes we want him to be able to do so, and sometimes we do not. We can nominally scale the items by presenting them to a subject and asking him which item he prefers, A or B? Are the two items different, yes or no? Which item is darker, has more luster, etc? The task is an easy one for the untrained evaluator. The response is simple and requires no reliance on memory. If an improvement or change in an item is thought to be small and if it is important to determine if a subject can see this difference between items, I suggest that the triangle test [*4*] be used. Items are presented to the subject three at a time; two are the same, one is different. The subject is asked to select the odd item. The advantage of the triangle test is that the judge's opportunity to guess correctly when he cannot detect a difference is reduced from one-half in a paired test to one-third.

The total number of trials and the number of times that a subject must make a correct decision before we can conclude that he can see a difference can be calculated prior to testing. This information is given for the paired and for the triangle test in Table 1.

"Difference" is the difference between A and B worth detecting. N is the number of pairs or triangles that a subject must evaluate; K equals the critical value. As an example, assume that it is important to be able to conclude that Fabrics A and B are different if the true difference is large enough to be detected 70 percent of the time. We would then choose a sample size of 63 paired comparisons. If a subject declares a difference 38 times or more, we conclude that he can see a difference between the two fabrics. If the difference is only commercially important when it is large, we might choose a sample size of 11 and be satisfied with detecting a difference only if it can be seen as often as 95 percent of the time. The critical value is calculated such that the probability of drawing a wrong conclusion is small, 0.05; that is, the probability of declaring a difference when there is none, and the probability of declaring that there is no difference when one exists does not exceed 5 percent. The table shows that fewer triads are needed than pairs to detect the same difference between items and that the subject must choose correctly less often. The N triads needed can be evaluated by N different people if you can assume that every subject can or cannot see the difference 100 percent of the time. The frequency of correct statements estimates the proportion of subjects who are sensitive to the degree of difference tested. Otherwise, N triads or pairs should be evaluated by each subject. The percentage of people who pick out the odd item K or more times estimates the degree of sensitivity of the population. *Biometrika* [5] or other statistical tables can be used to place 95 percent confidence limits on this estimate. One must then decide whether the proportion of people who can and cannot detect the difference is acceptable in an economic sense.

TABLE 1–*Sample size required to declare a difference between items A and B.*

Difference	Pairs			Triads		
%(A/B)	N	K	%(K)	N	K	%(K)
70	63	38	60	53	24	45
75	42	27	64	32	16	50
80	28	19	68	22	12	55
85	18	13	72	15	9	60
90	13	10	77	9	6	67
95	11	9	82	7	5	71

Example 1

This example was created to explain the triangle test. Standard paper was dyed by standard methods at standard strengths such that one sheet contained 100 parts of dye and one contained 105 parts of dye. This was done for each of two colors, blue and red. The sheets were cut into 2½-in. squares and placed onto an 8½ by 11-in. piece of paper such that the three items making up each triangle, two alike and one different, overlapped by an equal amount. Each of 91 subjects was asked to pick out the odd item in a total of 12 different trials for each color. The number of subjects choosing correctly in from 0 to 12 triads is plotted in Fig. 1.

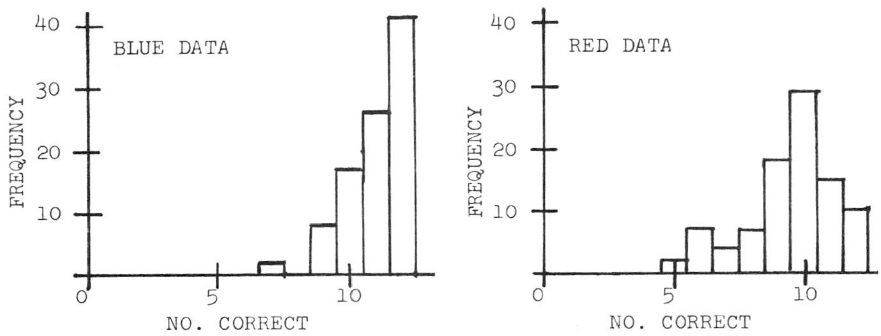

FIG. 1—*Triangle test—frequency of correct choices.*

We are confident that a subject can see the five-part difference if he chose the odd item 8 out of 12 times. The proportion of subjects that did is $\hat{p} = 0.98$ for blue and $\hat{p} = 0.86$ for red. $\hat{p}$ estimates the true proportion p. Ninety-five percent confidence limits on the estimates are

$$\Pr (0.93 \leqslant p \leqslant 1.00) = 0.95$$

$$\Pr (0.78 \leqslant p \leqslant 0.92) = 0.95$$

respectively. Note that the confidence limits do not overlap. This indicates that the two proportions are different. The red color decreases a subject's sensitivity to the dye difference.

Thresholds

Multiple triangle tests can be used to find subjective thresholds. Items are chosen to represent varying differences in dye levels. A triangle test is then run on each pair of items. Resulting data can be plotted as in Fig. 2.

The effectiveness of the triangle test may be product dependent. A subject in

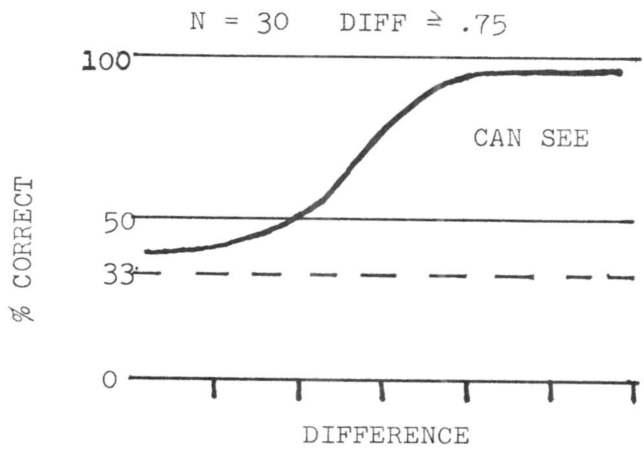

FIG. 2–*Smallest difference that can be observed.*

the experiment just mentioned thought that the overlapping edges of the triangles helped him to pick out the odd item more quickly. It is realistic, however, in dye studies where small differences may be objectionable to compare items at least side by side. Otherwise, an important matching problem may go unobserved. In most applications this problem does not occur. Coffees and other beverages and foods are tasted individually and can be given to the subject one at a time in a random order.

Ordinal Scaling

Most frequently when we desire to relate subjective responses to objective data, we are not interested in small item differences but wish to analytically predict over a wide range of subjective response. We obtain subjective data most easily by obtaining an ordinal scaling of items chosen to represent differences along the property of interest. The experiment is designed to obtain all relationships between items, directly or by inference. Ordinal scaling increases the task for the subject, but designs can be used such that a subject need not compare all items at one time. Balanced incomplete block designs [*6*] can be used, for example, to obtain a complete rank order of all items. The design given in Table 2 is a balanced incomplete block design (B.I.B.D.) of block size three for six items. The design is called balanced because every item appears equally often. It is called incomplete because all items are not compared at the same time. The design in Table 2 requires five samples of each item. Each pair is evaluated twice. If the items are small, the triples can be arranged on tables around a room. Each subject is asked to go from table to table choosing the item that has, say, the most luster and the item that has the least. A subject's

TABLE 2–*Example–B.I.B.D., six items, block size three.*

Triple No.	Items	Most	Least	Rank Item No.	Score
1	1 2 4	1	4	6	10
2	3 4 6	6	3	5	8
3	1 3 5	5	3	1	6
4	2 3 6	6	3	2	4
5	1 3 4	1	3	4	2
6	4 5 6	6	4	3	0
7	2 3 5	5	3		
8	1 5 6	6	1		
9	2 4 5	5	4		
10	1 2 6	6	2		

evaluations can be readily combined into one rank order in the manner given by H. A. David [*3*]. A score of 2.0 is given to the item declared to be most lustrous, a score of 0.0 is given to the item declared to be least lustrous, and a score of 1.0 is given to the third item in the triple. If these scores are summed for each item, the item score becomes the number of times that the item was declared to be more lustrous than all other items. The design can be replicated to obtain a better estimate of subject consistency. Three digit codes can be used to identify each item to deter subject recognition of an item previously evaluated. If all subjects agree on the rank order of the items, the scores for each item can be averaged across people. One score for each item is obtained, and the results can be used along with analytical measurements in correlation or regression analysis to describe the relationship between subjective and objective data [*7*]. If subjects do not agree, the data from groups of subjects with like opinions should be analyzed separately.

Items can be arranged in pairs instead of triples for evaluation. However, three times the number of pairs are needed to obtain the same information. Blocks of a larger size can also be used. If more than three items are evaluated at one time, the amount of effort required of the subject increases considerably.

Other Designs

If multiple samples of several or all of the items cannot be obtained or facilities are not available to collect data on many triples at once, B.I.B.D.'s are not the most efficient way to rank items.

One method by which all items can be ranked relatively easily at one time is what I call the "Cluster or Group Division" method of ranking. A description follows.

All items are placed on a table or other suitable device. The subject then splits the items into two piles. One pile contains those that are more lustrous than others and one contains those that are less lustrous. The subject keeps splitting the piles in a similar fashion until the items are completely ranked from most to least lustrous. An example is given in Table 3.

A subject should be allowed to check her rank order at completion since it is very easy to make a mistake early in grouping. The largest number of items that we have evaluated using this method is 40. The disadvantage of this scaling method compared to triples is that no measure of subject consistency is obtained unless the subject completely reranks the items. Triples or other B.I.B.D.'s provide a measure of consistency in the following manner. If a subject chooses Item A over Item B and Item B over Item C, she should logically choose Item A over Item C. If she chooses C over A instead, she is inconsistent. This event is called a circular triad. The number of circular triads can be compared to the number that we might expect for a person that has ranked the items randomly [*3*].

Improving Ordinal Data

A criticism of rank order data is that large and small differences obtain equal weight. One attempt to create a finer scale is called "Powering." This is discussed in Kendall's paper [*8*]. Basically, data is powered by giving the item declared to be "most lustrous" the sum of the scores of items declared to be less lustrous. The second most lustrous item is given the sum of the scores of items ranked below it, etc. This is done iteratively, normalizing the scores to keep them small, until further adjustments do not change the score values. Attempts have also been made to rate or rank differences between items [*1,2*].

Correlation Between Subjective and Objective

After the items have been subjectively scaled, we can attempt to find the relationship between the subjective rank order and one or more analytical measurements. A combination of analytical tests may best correlate with the subjective scaling. As stated earlier, common techniques utilize correlation and regression analyses. In cases where analytical variables are correlated, factor analysis, modified factor analysis, or ridge regression should be used [*9,10*]. If the analytical method can predict all but a few subjective points as shown in Fig. 3, we can study the subjective data to see if judges had difficulty in ranking

TABLE 3–*Example–cluster ranking, ten items.*

Less Lustrous	More Lustrous
[3,5,8,9]	[1,2,4,6,7,10]
[5,8] [3,9]	[1,2,4,10] [6,7]
Least 5 8 9 3	1 10 2 4 6 7 Most

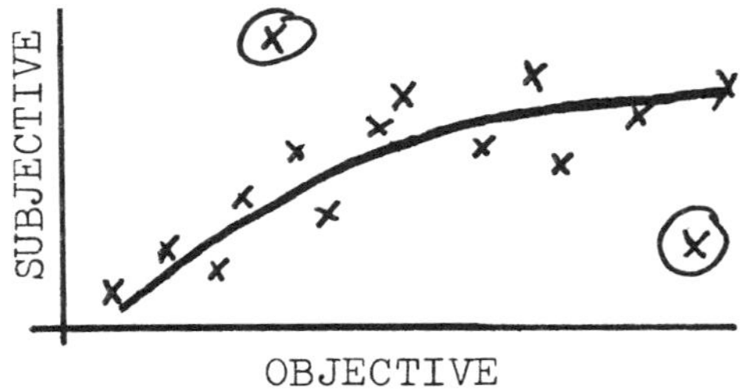

FIG. 3–*Illustration–relationship between objective and subjective data.*

those items. If this is confirmed, the triangle test can be used to see if the items are distinctly different from other items.

Example 2

This example was initiated to try to predict subjective impressions of the nonuniformity of full-fashioned sweater yarns. The goal was threefold; (1) to find the relationship between subjective impressions of uniformity and four analytical measurements, (2) to find the acceptable level of uniformity, and (3) to determine if greige or unfinished yarn could be tested instead of finished yarn. The yarns scaled were chosen to represent a range of uniformity. They differed in type, fiber denier, and textile processing route.

Design

Twenty judges ranked 15 full fashioned greige and finished sweater swatches from most to least uniform by the "Cluster Ranking" technique. Later, we realized that all or none of the yarns might be acceptable. We obtained 12 of the original judges to consider each item individually and declare it to be acceptable or unacceptable. Each subject evaluated all items twice.

Analysis

Correlation analysis showed that all judges, with one exception, agreed on the rank order or the two sets of items. Coefficients of correlation ranged from 0.80 to 0.95. A coefficient of 1.0 would represent perfect agreement. A coefficient of –1.0 would represent perfect disagreement. The data from the judge giving a different rank order were eliminated from further analysis. The remaining data were averaged into one rank order. The scores are given in Table 4.

TABLE 4—*Sweaters—rank order and average score.*

Greige			Finished		
Fabric No.	A.S.[a]	Average Score	Fabric No.	A.S.[a]	Average Score
1	24	13.5	1	24	13.8
2	20	12.1	4	13	12.5
4	22	11.9	3	13	11.5
3	17	11.2	2	10	11.0
7	10	9.8	5	10	9.6
5	13	8.2	7	7	9.2
6	4	8.0	11	4	6.3
8	0	7.2	6	3	6.2
10	4	5.9	8	2	5.5
11	2	5.2	10	2	4.9
9	1	3.9	14	2	4.6
12	1	3.3	9	3	4.2
14	1	1.8	13	0	2.8
13	1	1.7	15	4	1.7
15	2	1.2	12	1	1.3

[a] A.S. = Acceptance score. It is the number of times the fabric was declared to be acceptable.

Ranking

Most uniform	1	1
	2,4,3	4,3
	7	3,2
	5,6,8	5,7
	10,11	11,5,8
	9,12	8,10,14
	13,14,15	10,14,9
Least uniform		13,15
		15,12

Fabrics are ranked from most to least uniform. The difference between fabric scores should be checked to make sure that the fabrics are distinguishably different. Otherwise, an observed difference may occur by chance and the observed rank order may not be reproducible. In this study, each pair of fabrics was evaluated 38 times for uniformity and 24 times for acceptability. We conclude that a fabric is acceptable if it is declared as such in 16 out of 24 comparisons; binomial significance test[*3,5*]. We conclude that two fabrics are distinguishably different if the difference in the average rank score is 1.3 or larger, multiple range test[*11*].

Note that more items were considered to be acceptable as greige fabric than after they had been finished. Also the rank order of greige fabric is more distinct. The more uniform the greige fabric, the more uniform the finished fabric; coefficient of correlation of 0.94. Fabric finishing, however, appears to diminish the distinctness of nonuniformities.

Analytical Prediction

Analytical measures of the coefficient of variation (CV) and the number of lows, thicks, and neps which describe the type of uneveness in a yarn sample were taken on singles and plied yarn for each type of sweater yarn. They are given in Table 5.

TABLE 5–*Full fashion sweater yarns–analytical measurements.*

	Single Yarns				Plied Yarns			
Identity	%CV	Lows	Thicks	Neps	%CV	Lows	Thicks	Neps
1	11.5	22	3	15	8.5	0	0	8
2	12.0	82	0	19	9.5	1	0	20
3	12.5	94	5	19	9.7	4	4	31
4	13.4	163	6	19	9.9	2	3	21
5	14.3	160	11	31	10.5	3	1	25
6	15.5	200	21	150	10.5	2	1	60
7	15.7	1574	3	58	10.6	1	4	36
8	16.0	360	8	61	10.5	2	1	119
9	17.0	504	32	138	12.3	14	1	95
10	17.4	658	18	95	12.9	26	3	47
11	18.0	987	52	62	13.2	21	4	110
12	18.4	193	7	321	13.6	48	3	121
13	18.5	860	19	117	12.6	22	5	51
14	19.2	1230	73	65	13.6	65	4	26
15	20.4	2419	397	315	14.9	158	4	55

Coefficients of correlation show that percent CV is best correlated with subjective uniformity, Table 6. The lower the CV, the more uniform the fabric, Figure 4. Measurements on singles yarn correlate slightly better than those on plied yarn.

TABLE 6–*Coefficients of correlation–subjective versus analytical.*

	Singles				Plied			
Full Fashioned	% CV	Lows	Thicks	Neps	% CV	Lows	Thicks	Neps
Greige	−0.96	−0.59	−0.51	−0.68	−0.93	−0.67	−0.51	−0.50
Finished	−0.93	−0.80	−0.44	−0.50	−0.89	−0.61	−0.39	−0.65

A single linear equation describes the relationship between subjective uniformity and percent CV rather well. The amount of variation in the subjective response related to a change in singles percent CV is 86 percent for finished yarn and 92 percent for greige yarn.

$$\text{finished subjective uniformity} = 28.5 - 1.34 \text{ (percent CV singles)}$$
$$\text{greige subjective uniformity} = 29.8 - 1.43 \text{ (percent CV singles)}$$

A one-unit increase in percent CV corresponds to a 1.3-unit decrease in finished subjective uniformity and a 1.4-unit decrease in greige subjective uniformity.

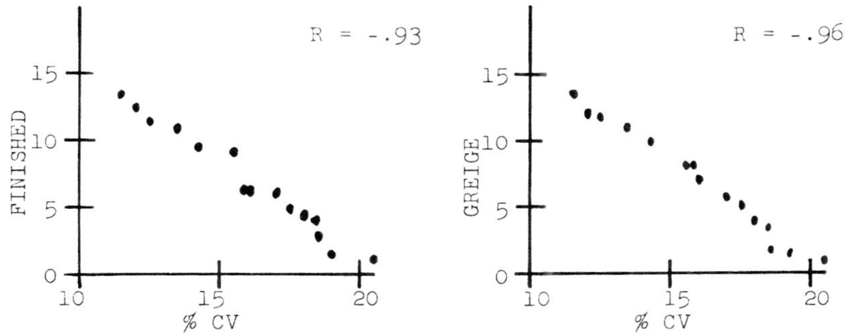

FIG. 4—*Correlation between percent CV and subjective uniformity scaling.*

Example 3

The last example is one in which all subjects do not agree upon product evaluation. The researcher was experimenting with finishes to whiten and to prevent the discoloration of men's shirting fabrics. He had three questions: (1) how do consumers define whiteness? (2) can we predict what they see analytically? The analytical predictor of interest was the Hunter D25 colorimeter, and (3) are the whitest shirts most preferred?

Design

The shirt fabric of interest was polyester. Fourteen fabrics were chosen for the evaluation. Some were new, some had been worn and washed one or more times. Some had been treated with tints, some had been bleached, and others had been scoured. The shirts were cut into swatches and evaluated in pairs, 91 pairs of 14 items. Each pair was evaluated twice. A subject was asked to choose the whitest shirt of the pair the first time that she saw the fabric. At a later time, she was asked to choose the fabric she preferred for whiteness. The fabrics were arranged on 28 tables around a room. Items were rearranged seven times to obtain all paired information.

Consistency

The paired data were combined into one rank order for each subject. Subject consistency can easily be checked by glancing at matices such as the one shown in Table 7 for Person 1.

The matrix represents the number of times that the row item was chosen over the column item. The row scores are summed to obtain the number of times that each fabric was chosen over all other fabrics. Each person had 91 chances of choosing the same item for whiteness; that is, 91 pairs evaluated twice. If Person 1 was perfectly consistent, the lower diagonal of the above matrix would be empty. She was able to repeat her comparisons 71 out of 91 times. The critical value, or minimum value to conclude consistency, is 54, binomial significance [*3,5*].

The sum of squares of row sum scores is also a measure of consistency. The higher the sum of squares, the more discriminating the subject. A plot of the frequency of each sum of squares, Figure 5, will show subjects who are more inconsistent than others. A critical value can also be calculated [*3*]. If the sum of squares for a subject exceeds the critical value, we can conclude that her data are distinguishably different from random data. The two right-hand columns in Table 7 show row sum scores for a subject that is perfectly consistent and for a subject that is perfectly inconsistent. Extreme inconsistency over all people indicates that the items are too similar for discrimination.

Subject Agreement

If subjects agree, we can combine their responses to obtain one rank order of all items. If not, we should separate the subjects into groups of people with like opinions. The percentage of people in each group estimates the proportion of the population that will prefer a particular item or market share.

The degree to which subjects rated the items in a similar manner was assessed through rank correlation [*12*]. Some women were highly correlated; others were not. Subjects can be rapidly separated into groups of subjects that rank in a similar manner with high speed computation and clustering techniques. I use the max method of S. C. Johnson [*13*] to find compact clusters of subjects. Correlation coefficients between all subjects can be used as input to the computer program, or the row sum data can be used. If row sum data are used, the computer program calculates the distance between all pairs of subjects. The two subjects with the shortest distance, or best agreement, are combined in the first iteration. The computer then searches for the next smallest distance. The new item that will be combined with an existing cluster is the one that has the minimum of the maximum distances between that cluster and all other items. An illustration is given in Figure 6.

TABLE 7–*Person 1–whiteness, data summary.*

ITEM	6	2	7	4	5	8	1	10	14	11	13	3	12	9	Row Sum Score	Perfectly Consistent	Inconsistent
6	. . .	1	2	2	2	2	2	2	2	2	2	2	2	2	25	26	13
2	1	. . .	2	2	2	1	2	2	2	2	2	2	0	2	22	24	13
7	0	0	. . .	1	2	2	2	1	2	2	1	2	2	2	19	22	13
4	0	0	1	. . .	2	2	0	2	1	2	2	2	2	2	18	20	13
5	0	0	0	0	. . .	1	2	2	2	2	2	2	2	2	17	18	13
8	0	1	0	0	1	. . .	0	1	2	2	1	2	2	2	14	16	13
1	0	0	0	2	0	2	. . .	1	1	1	1	0	1	2	11	14	13
10	0	0	1	0	0	1	1	. . .	1	1	1	2	2	2	12	12	13
14	0	0	0	1	0	0	1	1	. . .	1	2	2	2	2	12	10	13
11	0	0	0	0	0	0	1	1	1	. . .	2	2	1	2	10	8	13
13	0	0	1	0	0	1	1	1	0	0	. . .	1	2	2	9	6	13
3	0	0	0	0	0	0	2	0	0	0	1	. . .	2	2	7	4	13
12	0	2	0	0	0	0	1	0	0	1	0	0	. . .	2	6	2	13
9	0	0	0	0	0	0	0	0	0	0	0	0	0	. . .	0	0	13
									No. 2's: 71 out of 91					Sum	182	182	182
									No. 1's: 40					Sum Squares	2954	3276	2366

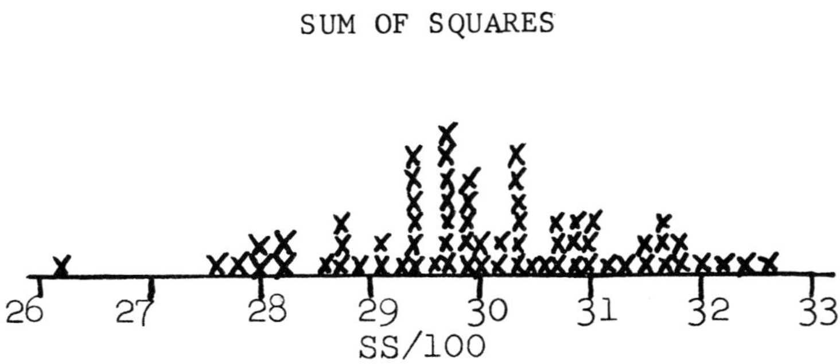

FIG. 5–*Subject consistency.*

Cluster:

Persons A and B
Is C or D next?
$d_2 > d_1$, therefore C = d_2
$d_4 > d_3$, therefore D = d_4
$d_4 > d_2$, therefore C is joined.

where

$$d_1 = \sqrt{(X_{B_1} - X_{C_1})^2 + (X_{B_2} - X_{C_2})^2 + \ldots + (X_{B_{14}} - X_{C_{14}})^2}\text{, and}$$

X_{B_1} = Person B's score for Item 1.

Iteration is discontinued when the next iteration combines clusters whose distance is large compared to the distances between subjects within a cluster.

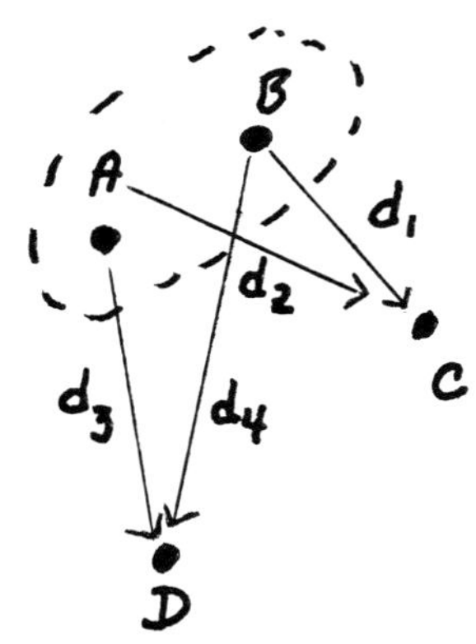

FIG. 6–*Illustration of cluster method.*

The cluster analysis of whiteness data gave three clusters of women who ranked the items similarly. Row sum scores were combined within each cluster. A summary of the results are given in Table 8. Item 9, a commercial item which had been scoured, was one of the least preferred. Item 6, a candidate textone bleached item, was one of the most. Clearly, Item 6 would be chosen as the one that would satisfy the majority of the ladies. Items 6 and 7 are identical except for an antistatic finish on Fabric 6. Item 1 is perceived differently by Cluster 1. Item 2 is perceived differently by all three clusters.

Correlation Between Preference and Whiteness

Subjects prefer items that they consider whitest. Coefficients of correlation between whiteness and preference data are 0.98 for Cluster 1, 0.99 for Cluster 2, and 0.96 for Cluster 3. Fabric 6 was preferred by all women. Fabric 9 was one of the least preferred.

Subjective Response versus Objective Measurements

Hunter D25 L, A, B, and W readings were taken on each shirt fabric with and without ultraviolet light. The coefficients of correlation between subjective whiteness and Hunter D25 readings are given in Table 9. In general, ultraviolet include readings correlate better with subjective whiteness than ultraviolet exclude.

W-IN measures subjective whiteness for the largest cluster of women quite well. B-IN and W-EX do nearly as well. No analytical reading, however, correlates well enough to expect a good relationship for Cluster 2.

A weighted sum of L,A,B include ratings relates as well as or better than any single reading for all subjective groups. The weighting must be done with some care because the analytical readings themselves are correlated. Correlation coefficients between the weighted sum and each cluster are 0.92, 0.89, and 0.95, respectively. The weighting shown in Table 10 is different for each group.

These weightings can be studied to determine differences between clusters. W is an integrated measure of whiteness. B measures blueness, blue (−) to yellow (+). A measures pinkness, green (−) to red (+). L measures brightness, black (0) to white (100 percent). We can compare the relative weight of each color scale regardless of the difference in the number size of L, A, and B values by looking at the correlation-based regression weights[*9*] given in Table 11.

People in Cluster 1 choose blue-white shirts as whitest more frequently than do the others. Clusters 2 and 3 are more affected by lightness. Cluster 2 also chooses pink-white shirts more frequently than do the others.

Summary

In summary, I have described and shown how certain sets of tools are interrelated to assess and define the relationship between objective measure-

TABLE 8–*Rank order of fabrics for whiteness.*

Cluster 1 (38 Women)		Cluster 2 (16 Women)		Cluster 3 (12 Women)	
Item	Score	Item	Score	Item	Score
Whitest					
2	22.6	6	24.7	6	24.1
6,4,1	20.9,20.7,20.0	7	19.9	7,10	19.7,18.1
5	18.8	4,5	16.7	8,13,12,3,11,5,14	15.0,14.2,13.9,13.7,13.3, 13.0,12.7
7	16.0	8,2,10	14.7,14.2,14.2		
8	14.6	11,13,14,3	11.6,10.6,10.3,10.1	11,5,14,4	13.3,13.0,12.7,11.1
14,11	10.7	13,14,3,12	10.6,10.3,10.1,9.2	2,9	6.1
10,13	8.5,7.7	1	6.4	1	1.0
3	5.9	9	2.3		
12	4.6				
9	0.4				
Least White					
Multiple range test Critical value					
	1.3		2.1		2.4

NOTE–Items appearing on the same line are not distinguishably different. Items that have the same score appear on the same line opposite one score.

TABLE 9–*Coefficients of correlation–subjective versus Hunter.*

	W-EX	W-IN	B-EX	B-IN	A-EX	A-IN	L-IN
Cluster 1	0.89	0.93	−0.79	−0.89	−0.21	0.40	−0.47
Cluster 2	0.31	0.53	−0.07	−0.32	0.32	0.64	0.34
Cluster 3	−0.36	−0.07	0.58	0.33	0.56	0.47	0.86

TABLE 10–*Explanation of cluster whiteness–weighted sum.*

	Constant	B-IN	A-IN	L-IN	R
Cluster 1	−28.2	−2.00	3.36	0.336	0.85
Cluster 2	−176.6	−1.44	3.95	1.97	0.78
Cluster 3	−245.5	−0.761	2.13	2.76	0.91

TABLE 11–*Correlation–based weights.*

	B-IN	A-IN	L-IN
Cluster 1	−0.885	0.238	0.108
Cluster 2	−0.794	0.350	0.795
Cluster 3	−0.406	0.182	1.07

ments and subjective responses. Although these tools can be used to assess the relationship for a variety of products or properties, the goals of each study should be clearly defined, and the study should be carefully planned. Other techniques may be more appropriate or more sensitive for a particular study, and logistic considerations may require modifications.

Acknowledgment

D. H. Doehlert designed and provided the first analysis for the example on the whiteness of men's shirting fabric. He also provided the design and obtained the colors for the example that was used to explain the triangle test.

References

[1] Doehlert, D. H. in *Basic Principles of Sensory Evaluation, ASTM STP 433,* American Society for Testing and Materials, 1968, pp. 58-78.

[2] Torgerson, W. S., *Theory and Methods of Scaling,* Wiley, New York, 1958.

[3] David, H. A., "The Method of Paired Comparisons," *Griffins Statistical Monographs and Courses,* No. 12, Hafner, New York, 1963.

[4] Ura, Shoji, "Pair, Triangle, Duo-Trio Test," Reports of Statistical Applications, Research 7, Japanese Union of Scientists and Engineers, 1960.

[5] Pearson, E. S. and Hartley, H. O., *Biometrika Tables for Statisticians,* Vol. I, Cambridge University Press, New York, 1956.

[6] Cochran, W. G. and Cox, G. M., *Experimental Designs,* Wiley, New York, 1957.
[7] Draper, N. R. and Smith, H., *Applied Regression Analysis,* Wiley, New York, 1966.
[8] Kendall, M. G. *Biometrics,* 1955, p. 11.
[9] Gollob, H. F., *Psychometrika,* 1968, p. 33.
[10] Hoerl, A. E. and Kennard, R. W., *Technometrics,* Vol. 12, No. 1, 1970.
[11] Starks, T. H. and David, H. A., "Significance Tests for Paired Comparison Experiments," *Biometrika,* 1961.
[12] Siegel, S., *Nonparametric Statistics,* McGraw-Hill, New York, 1956.
[13] Johnson, S. C., "Hierarchical Clustering Schemes," *Psychometrics,* 1967.

Myron Wish[1] *and J. Douglas Carroll*[1]

Concepts and Applications of Multidimensional Scaling

REFERENCE: Wish, Myron and Carroll, J. Douglas, "**Concepts and Applications of Multidimensional Scaling,**" *Sensory Evaluation of Appearance of Materials, ASTM STP 545,* American Society for Testing and Materials, 1973, pp. 91-108.

ABSTRACT: Multidimensional scaling (MDS) is a general term for a class of techniques that can be used to develop spatial representations of psychological stimuli or other objects. The typical input data for these procedures is a matrix of distance-like numbers which indicate how similar or different every stimulus is to each of the others. These similarity or dissimilarity values may be based on objective measurements or subjective judgments. MDS techniques involve iterative algorithms, usually requiring high-speed computers, for constructing the spatial configuration, or "map."

Although some mention is made of earlier MDS procedures, primary attention is given to describing and illustrating a new technique called "INDSCAL," for INdividual Differences SCALing. The input to INDSCAL is several matrices of similarities or dissimilarities among the objects, usually one for each subject participating in a study. The output from INDSCAL includes information about the weight, or perceptual importance, of each dimension for every subject, as well as a multidimensional space for the stimulus objects. The applications illustrate the wide range of stimuli and experimental methods that can be used in studies involving MDS, and demonstrate some special advantages of INDSCAL.

KEY WORDS: senses, perception, dimensional analysis, scale (ratio), stimulus (psychophysiology), measurement

Multidimensional scaling (MDS) is a general term for a class of techniques that can be used to develop spatial representations of psychological stimuli or other objects. These techniques involve iterative algorithms, usually requiring high-speed computers, for constructing the spatial configuration, or "map." The typical data used in an MDS analysis is one or more matrices of distance-like numbers, based on objective measurements or psychological judgments. We shall use the term "proximities" *[1-3]*[2] to refer to any such set of distance-like

[1] Members of Technical Staff, Bell Laboratories, Inc., Murray Hill, N. J. 07974.

[2] The italic numbers in brackets refer to the list of references appended to this paper.

numbers. (In some cases the proximities are directly related to spatial distances, while in others they are inversely related.) MDS procedures determine the dimensions relevant to the perception of the stimuli and locate the stimulus objects on each dimension of the resulting space. Distances between points in the multidimensional space reflect, as well as statistically possible, the proximities of the associated stimuli.

In the earlier metric MDS procedures [*4*], the proximities were assumed to be linearly related to distances in the underlying space. Shepard [*1*] made an important breakthrough in the area of nonmetric MDS. His computerized procedure required only that the proximities reflect the rank order of the distances. Kruskal [*5,6*] developed and computerized a nonmetric MDS program, called M-D-SCAL, which perfected the rationale of Shepard's procedure and introduced important improvements.

Some Basic Concepts of Multidimensional Scaling

Perhaps the simplest way to explain what MDS does is to show how it could be used to reconstruct a map from a table of airline distances. Figure 1*B* shows such a table. The proximity value in row *i* and column *j* of this table, or matrix, is the actual airline distance between cities *i* and *j*. It is a simple matter to construct this airline distance table from the map in Fig. 1*A;* one measures the distance between each pair of cities with a ruler and converts these distances to miles by means of the scale shown in the lower left-hand corner.

The reverse problem of reconstructing the map from the table of distances is much more difficult to do by hand, particularly if there is considerable random error in the data and if more than two dimensions are needed. This is where MDS comes in—that is, it provides an efficient way to develop a spatial representation of any matrix of distances or distance-like numbers.

Figure 1*C* shows the two-dimensional space derived from the table of airline distances by means of Kruskal's [*5,6*] M-D-SCAL computer program. The program "instructed" the computer to find locations for each city (a stimulus) in a two-dimensional configuration such that the distances in the resulting space (computed by the Euclidean distance formula) would agree as well as possible with the original data values (Fig. 1*B*).

Since distances are unaffected by a rotation of the axes of the space, the dimensions from M-D-SCAL and most other MDS procedures are generally not in the most appropriate orientation. It is therefore usually necessary to rotate the axes to interpret, or make sense out of, the dimensions. Interpretation generally involves distinguishing how stimuli on one extreme of the dimension differ from those at the other extreme. This rotational problem is simple in two dimensions, but becomes prohibitively difficult as the number of dimensions increases. Of course, rotation presented no problems in this example since we knew exactly what to look for. The dimensions in this space are exactly what

(A) GEOGRAPHIC LOCATIONS OF TEN U.S. CITIES

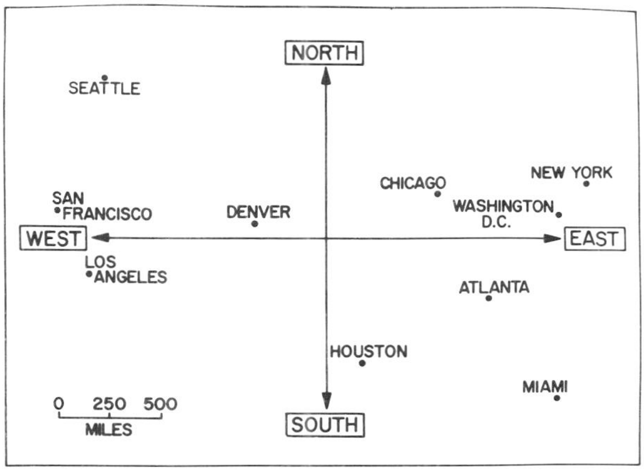

(B) AIRLINE DISTANCES BETWEEN TEN U.S. CITIES

CITIES	ATLA.	CHIC.	DENV.	HOUS.	L.A.	MIAMI	N.Y.	S.F.	SEAT.	WASH. D.C.
ATLANTA		587	1212	701	1936	604	748	2139	2182	543
CHICAGO	587		920	940	1745	1188	713	1858	1737	597
DENVER	1212	920		879	831	1726	1631	949	1021	1494
HOUSTON	701	940	879		1374	968	1420	1645	1891	1220
LOS ANGELES	1936	1745	831	1374		2339	2451	347	959	2300
MIAMI	604	1188	1726	968	2339		1092	2594	2734	923
NEW YORK	748	713	1631	1420	2451	1092		2571	2408	205
SAN FRANCISCO	2139	1858	949	1645	347	2594	2571		678	2442
SEATTLE	2182	1737	1021	1891	959	2734	2408	678		2329
WASHINGTON D.C.	543	597	1494	1220	2300	923	205	2442	2329	

(C) MD-SCAL SPACE FOR DISTANCES BETWEEN CITIES

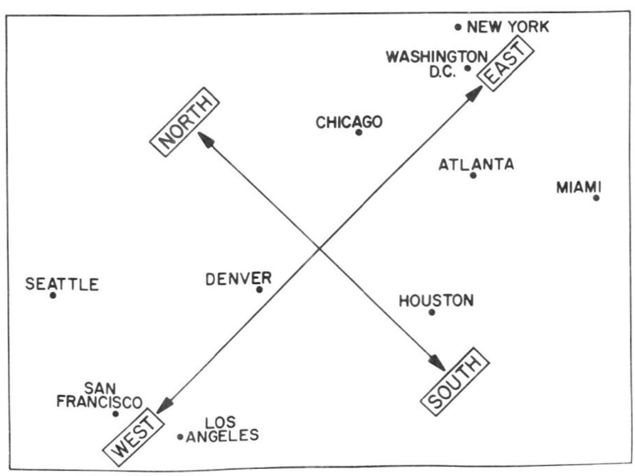

FIG. 1–*The airline distances between the ten U.S. cities in the map* (A), *are indicated in the matrix shown in* (B). *An M-D-SCAL*[5,6] *analysis of the matrix of airline distances produced the two-dimensional space in* (C). *It was necessary to rotate the axes of the space to get the appropriate orientation of the "North-South" and "East-West" dimensions.*

one would expect; namely, "North-South" and "East-West." (See Ref *7* for a discussion of statistical procedures which can be used for interpretations of dimensions.)

Figure 2 shows the degree of correspondence between the original data (Fig. 1*B*) and the derived distances (measured in Fig. 1*C*). There is a point for every pair of cities in this scatter diagram. The projection of a point on the vertical axis is equal to the airline distance specified in the table; the projection on the horizontal axis corresponds to the distance between the cities in the MDS space. Although there is a linear relationship for these data, M-D-SCAL allows for any monotonic or order-preserving function. The goodness (or badness) of fit is indicated by the extent of horizontal deviation of the points from the indicated function. Kruskal [*5,6*] uses an index called "stress" (which is a normalized residual sum of squares) to measure the total discrepancy. In fact, the goal of the procedure is to minimize the stress value (using the numerical method of steepest descent, or gradients) in the specified dimensionality. The stress for these data is 0.007, indicating an almost perfect fit.

A poor stress value generally means that there is considerable error in the data (as often occurs when subjective measures of proximity are used) or that more

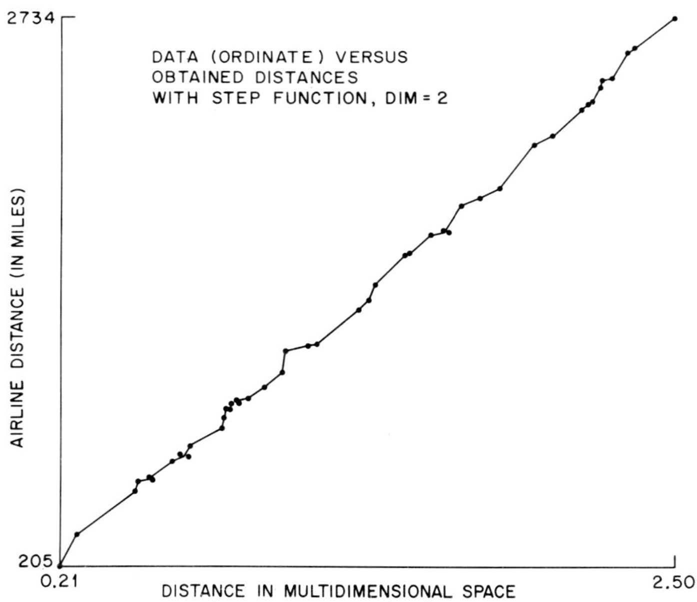

FIG. 2–*Scatter plot of airline distance data from Fig. 1*B *(Y-axis) vs distances in the two-dimensional space in Fig. 1*C*, derived from the data by Kruskal's M-D-SCAL procedure (X-axis).*

dimensions are needed. The most common procedure for estimating how many dimensions are appropriate for the data is to do MDS analyses in several dimensionalities, and to observe where the stress value starts to level off. For example, if the stress in three dimensions is much lower than in two, and if the stress of the four-dimensional solution is only slightly lower than that of the three-dimensional solution, one would probably conclude that only three dimensions are needed. In general, it is desirable to include as few dimensions as possible in order to get a parsimonious description of the data. However, one should also consider whether an extra dimension is interpretable and whether it adds insight into the data when deciding how many dimensions are appropriate.

In the example we have just discussed, the MDS analysis provided no new information about the data; it merely demonstrated that the underlying structure in a data matrix could be recovered by MDS. In most applications, however, we do not know what the dimensions are and how many there will be. Therefore, it takes foresight and skill to design the study in the first place and to use MDS effectively for analyzing the data. Of course, the benefits of MDS are much greater when the results are not known *a priori*, since one can learn a lot about the stimulus structure that would be almost impossible to discover by "eyeballing" the data matrix. This is not to say that MDS will reveal everything; rather, it provides valuable information which can be supplemented by other kinds of data analyses.

Some Methods for Collecting Proximities Data

There are many data collection methods that can be used to obtain measures of proximity between stimuli [*2,3,8*]. Some of these will be described briefly in order to illustrate the variety of data appropriate for MDS.

Perhaps the most common procedure used in psychology for getting proximities data is to ask subjects to give direct ratings of the degree of similarity between stimuli. In this regard, Fig. 3 shows a page from a questionnaire booklet in which subjects rated the degree of similarity between pairs of nations. These similarities can be assumed to be inversely related to distances, since higher similarity values reflect smaller psychological distance between nations. There are other variants of this kind of format; for example, one stimulus could appear at the top of the page, followed by a list of the remaining stimuli. In this method, judgments are usually made with respect to each of the stimuli; that is, each stimulus serves as a standard, appearing at the top of a different page. With visual stimuli it is often more convenient to give the subjects stimulus cards or even the objects themselves, and to ask the subjects for a similarity rating. Auditory stimuli frequently require special apparatus designed to present the stimuli; for example, see Bricker et al [*9*] and Pruzansky [*10*].

When there is a large number of stimuli to evaluate (more than 25 or 30) the

	DEGREE OF SIMILARITY								
	VERY DIFFERENT								VERY SIMILAR
1. A. CHINA (MAINLAND) B. EGYPT	1	2	3	4	5	6	7	8	9
2. A. RUSSIA (U.S.S.R.) B. INDIA	1	2	3	4	5	6	7	8	9
3. A. JAPAN B. RUSSIA (U.S.S.R.)	1	2	3	4	5	6	7	8	9
4. A. CONGO B. ISRAEL	1	2	3	4	5	6	7	8	9
5. A. INDIA B. YUGOSLAVIA	1	2	3	4	5	6	7	8	9
6. A. BRAZIL B. INDIA	1	2	3	4	5	6	7	8	9
7. A. EGYPT B. CONGO	1	2	3	4	5	6	7	8	9
8. A. ISRAEL B. JAPAN	1	2	3	4	5	6	7	8	9
9. A. CUBA B. BRAZIL	1	2	3	4	5	6	7	8	9
10. A. YUGOSLAVIA B. CUBA	1	2	3	4	5	6	7	8	9

FIG. 3—*Page from a questionnaire booklet in which subjects recorded their judgments of similarities between 12 nations* (*see Ref* 16).

number of pairs may be too great for a single subject to make all comparisons. In this case one can present different subsets of stimuli to different people. Another alternative, which is especially useful for exploratory studies, is to ask subjects to sort the stimuli into mutually exclusive and exhaustive categories so that stimuli in the same category are more similar to each other than to those in other categories. When such a sorting method is used, one typically derives an aggregate proximity matrix for the whole group or for various subgroups of subjects. The number of times each pair of stimuli is placed in the same category can then be used as the proximity measure (see also Rosenberg et al [*11*]).

There are ways to get indirect measures of proximity that are useful when dealing with visual, auditory, or other sensory stimuli. For example, one can present stimuli pairwise to subjects, and ask them to indicate whether the stimuli of each pair are the "same" or "different." Figure 4 shows a matrix of "confusions" among Morse Code-like signals derived from such a task[*12*]. These signals differ from the three component signals of the International Morse Code only in that the intervals between the dots and dashes can be long, like dashes (indicated by a 3), as well as short like dots (indicated by a 1). The value in row *i* and column *j* indicates the proportion of subjects who responded "same" to the pair in which stimulus *i* was presented first and stimulus *j* second. Although the matrix is not perfectly symmetric, there is a strong tendency for the *i,j* and *j,i* cells to be reasonably close in value. The diagonal cells, which correspond to correct responses, are much larger than most of the off-diagonal values, which indicate the errors, or confusions. (see Ref *13* for a discussion of desirable properties of a proximity matrix.)

Similar to the preceding method is one in which a single stimulus at a time is presented to subjects whose task it is to identify what they heard or saw (see Ref

		S_1	U_1	R_1	D_1	W_1	K_1	G_1	C_1	S_2	U_2	R_2	D_2	W_2	K_2	G_2	O_2	S_3	U_3	R_3	D_3	W_3	K_3	G_3	O_3	S_4	U_4	R_4	D_4	W_4	K_4	G_4	O_4	
·1·1·	S_1	97	94	81	66	16	31	06	03	79	18	28	11	01	04	02	01	44	11	05	01	00	02	01	02	02	02	00	00	00	01	03	02	S_1
·1·1-	U_1	63	98	86	74	91	73	23	16	57	61	49	21	13	09	06	00	44	35	06	08	04	07	03	01	03	00	03	03	05	01	00	02	U_1
·1-1·	R_1	27	73	94	50	72	62	51	22	42	52	64	49	30	11	16	00	23	22	33	22	14	12	12	04	07	07	12	09	01	05	02	09	R_1
-1·1·	D_1	47	75	69	96	33	94	67	09	43	13	40	34	11	26	19	02	28	16	17	50	00	05	03	06	03	02	00	07	03	02	04	00	D_1
·1-1-	W_1	03	40	64	42	94	76	68	70	20	51	73	40	69	49	54	31	22	33	25	17	31	18	12	08	09	19	19	11	06	09	06	00	W_1
-1·1-	K_1	07	44	33	69	69	95	70	67	19	37	40	56	26	74	27	16	08	27	32	47	17	46	11	08	03	06	05	16	06	06	01	01	K_1
-1-1·	G_1	01	08	49	50	78	78	93	82	08	14	48	80	23	53	90	33	04	11	47	37	40	27	22	38	10	18	19	38	13	14	11	06	G_1
-1-1-	O_1	02	10	19	04	31	51	76	97	00	04	12	16	20	50	82	82	05	11	25	09	38	31	23	57	11	31	08	33	31	28	14	09	O_1
·1·3·	S_2	44	54	62	56	32	41	19	04	94	84	62	54	38	22	07	00	69	45	27	39	10	21	06	01	25	11	03	17	00	00	02	02	S_2
·1·3-	U_2	03	39	44	15	66	61	29	19	63	94	39	52	77	48	14	07	30	45	22	24	21	34	09	14	20	27	03	08	04	15	05	03	U_2
·1-3·	R_2	05	16	48	15	59	19	45	28	31	38	95	47	86	36	53	12	19	25	33	24	33	19	21	07	10	14	27	32	11	02	06	01	R_2
-1·3·	D_2	06	14	28	46	26	51	69	43	47	39	43	94	35	79	73	35	09	18	34	42	15	37	33	16	19	17	19	51	05	34	09	00	D_2
·1-3-	W_2	02	14	24	09	62	39	2/	59	07	54	69	37	94	64	56	41	05	21	19	19	44	29	19	34	04	22	06	13	14	19	03	11	W_2
-1·3-	K_2	01	03	05	07	22	54	37	56	14	19	23	68	48	98	47	72	03	18	14	25	14	33	41	37	01	06	06	31	15	37	18	07	K_2
-1-3·	G_2	01	05	10	08	30	28	71	73	08	07	46	57	44	42	93	71	01	10	27	08	36	23	59	50	05	11	32	54	21	44	57	19	G_2
-1-3-	O_2	00	01	04	03	21	08	35	80	00	04	07	24	55	58	58	94	02	06	07	03	19	14	25	60	02	15	11	31	47	41	57	56	O_2
·3·1·	S_3	42	38	50	48	23	22	19	06	69	53	31	33	09	03	05	01	94	91	59	54	16	45	03	05	47	13	12	27	02	03	02	00	S_3
·3·1-	U_3	04	09	30	18	42	52	35	29	30	29	14	21	30	22	05	05	56	94	53	57	64	67	23	12	17	34	19	15	18	16	02	03	U_3
·3-1·	R_3	05	05	43	08	22	24	38	20	10	17	40	31	28	31	24	05	29	53	94	52	84	43	62	55	27	37	65	27	19	30	11	03	R_3
-3·1·	D_3	01	04	06	26	09	47	31	05	19	36	21	51	06	19	21	04	30	36	35	94	16	97	47	20	16	05	07	60	01	15	05	01	D_3
·3-1-	W_3	01	02	15	02	32	12	37	50	04	16	21	08	36	29	53	34	14	51	72	19	94	31	56	76	15	60	41	44	51	49	29	31	W_3
-3·1-	K_3	02	04	06	11	14	61	18	27	02	26	13	22	13	28	17	09	17	56	13	80	13	97	79	68	03	09	08	46	06	67	12	02	K_3
-3-1·	G_3	01	07	03	05	07	29	43	14	01	05	04	27	13	16	37	42	05	11	56	68	58	57	96	89	04	12	22	60	21	45	52	17	G_3
-3-1-	O_3	00	00	03	00	08	18	19	64	02	03	09	07	17	22	20	52	01	10	36	28	29	50	74	97	02	15	14	49	27	73	69	56	O_3
·3·3·	S_4	02	05	04	02	06	05	06	12	28	17	15	28	07	07	23	08	44	55	57	19	28	12	19	15	96	78	59	47	08	35	36	03	S_4
·3·3-	U_4	06	01	04	06	12	17	22	26	04	14	20	13	19	29	35	26	04	52	50	12	59	26	19	44	45	97	55	28	67	64	13	13	U_4
·3-3·	R_4	02	01	10	02	16	07	20	17	03	06	49	23	21	17	39	30	04	17	66	21	45	06	44	54	31	29	94	48	61	31	61	05	R_4
-3·3·	D_4	01	03	07	06	13	05	28	33	01	05	07	28	06	19	22	25	03	25	16	67	25	52	78	67	26	42	30	97	31	83	60	03	D_4
·3-3-	W_4	00	02	03	02	06	06	22	33	01	03	14	06	38	09	42	54	03	05	19	08	56	12	38	69	25	46	55	50	93	59	65	74	W_4
-3·3-	K_4	01	01	00	02	02	07	05	32	01	05	02	10	11	27	28	34	04	08	06	28	15	75	56	83	06	42	15	81	16	98	37	53	K_4
-3-3·	G_4	01	01	01	01	06	06	26	18	02	03	07	01	08	11	59	47	00	03	11	07	27	08	74	80	05	22	35	62	33	55	97	51	G_4
-3-3-	O_4	00	02	00	01	00	01	07	09	02	01	00	02	06	05	35	64	03	01	00	01	06	03	26	89	06	09	17	05	42	53	75	97	O_4
		S_1	U_1	R_1	D_1	W_1	K_1	G_1	O_1	S_2	U_2	R_2	D_2	W_2	K_2	G_2	O_2	S_3	U_3	R_3	D_3	W_3	K_3	G_3	O_3	S_4	U_4	R_4	D_4	W_4	K_4	G_4	O_4	

FIG. 4–*Matrix of perceptual confusions among 32 three-component Morse Code-like signals*[12]. *The* 1's *and* 3's *between the dots and dashes indicate whether the intercomponent interval is short (of dot-length) or long (of dash-length). The signals were presented pair-wise to 324 subjects who judged whether the signals of the pair were the "same" or "different." The cell values indicate the percentage of "same" responses for each ordered pair of signals (row signal preceded column signal).*

14). The proportion of presentations of stimulus *i* in which the response *j* is given may be used as a measure of the proximity between stimulus *i* and stimulus *j*. These confusion methods, of course, require that the stimuli not be so discriminable that no errors are made, nor so confusable that no stimulus can be discriminated from another. It is, therefore, usually necessary to degrade the stimuli in some way (such as by adding noise or by presenting the stimuli tachistoscopically at a fast rate) to attain the desired level of discriminability.

Another common way to get proximities data is to compute some measure of similarity or dissimilarity between profiles of pairs of stimuli. These profiles can be based on objective measurements, such as height and weight, or on subjective ratings of the stimuli. For example, political scientists and economists have often derived measures of proximity between nations from indices such as gross national product, population, standard of living, etc. The proximity measure could be the correlation between rows or columns of the table, or some measure of profile dissimilarity such as the D^2-measure (see Refs *11* and *15*). Although correlational data derived from profiles of objective or subjective data have typically been analyzed by factor-analytic or clustering procedures, such data are also appropriate input for MDS.

There are many other data-collection procedures that can be used to get measures of proximity between stimuli. However, the preceding discussion should suffice to give an idea of the range of methods that can be used in MDS studies.

An Application of M-D-SCAL to Data on Nation Perceptions

The next example shows that MDS can reveal a lot about the structure in a data matrix that was not known in advance. The data is from a pilot study conducted in 1968 on perceptions of nations [*16,17*]. In the experimental task under discussion, 18 Columbia University students (in a class taught by the first author) rated the degree of similarity between 12 nations. The format of the response booklet in which subjects recorded their judgments has already been illustrated (Fig. 3). Figure 5 shows the matrix of averaged ratings for nations; that is, the value in each cell is the average rating of similarity for that pair of nations by the 18 students. This matrix was used as input to Kruskal's [*5,6*] M-D-SCAL computer program.

The two-dimensional solution is displayed in Fig. 6. As indicated in the figure, it was necessary to rotate the axes to interpret the dimensions. The dimension going from the upper left to the lower right of the space distinguishes the Communist from the Non-Communist countries, with the neutral countries in between; the dimension going from the lower left to the upper right orders nations according to their economic development. Although the goodness-of-fit measure gave some suggestion that a third dimension was needed (the stress, using Stress Formula 1, in two dimensions was 0.187), no satisfactory

	1 BR	2 CO	3 CU	4 EG	5 FR	6 IN	7 IS	8 JA	9 CH	10 RU	11 US	12 YU
1. Brazil	---	4.8	5.3	3.4	4.7	4.5	3.8	3.5	2.4	3.1	5.4	3.2
2. Congo	4.8	---	4.6	5.0	4.0	4.8	3.3	3.4	4.0	3.4	2.4	3.5
3. Cuba	5.3	4.6	---	5.2	4.1	4.0	3.6	2.9	5.5	5.4	3.2	5.1
4. Egypt	3.4	5.0	5.2	---	4.8	5.8	4.7	3.8	4.4	4.4	3.3	4.3
5. France	4.7	4.0	4.1	4.8	---	3.4	4.0	4.2	3.7	5.1	5.9	4.7
6. India	4.5	4.8	4.0	5.8	3.4	---	4.1	4.5	4.1	4.5	4.3	4.0
7. Israel	3.8	3.3	3.6	4.7	4.0	4.1	---	4.8	3.0	4.2	5.9	4.4
8. Japan	3.5	3.4	2.9	3.8	4.2	4.5	4.8	---	4.2	4.6	6.1	4.3
9. China (Mainland)	2.4	4.0	5.5	4.4	3.7	4.1	3.0	4.2	---	5.7	2.6	5.1
10. Russia	3.1	3.4	5.4	4.4	5.1	4.5	4.2	4.6	5.7	---	5.0	6.7
11. U.S.A.	5.4	2.4	3.2	3.3	5.9	4.3	5.9	6.1	2.6	5.0	---	3.6
12. Yugoslavia	3.2	3.5	5.1	4.3	4.7	4.0	4.4	4.3	5.1	6.7	3.6	---

FIG. 5.–*Matrix of averaged ratings* (N = *18*) *of similarity between 12 nations* (*on a scale from* 1, *for very different, to* 9, *for very similar*).

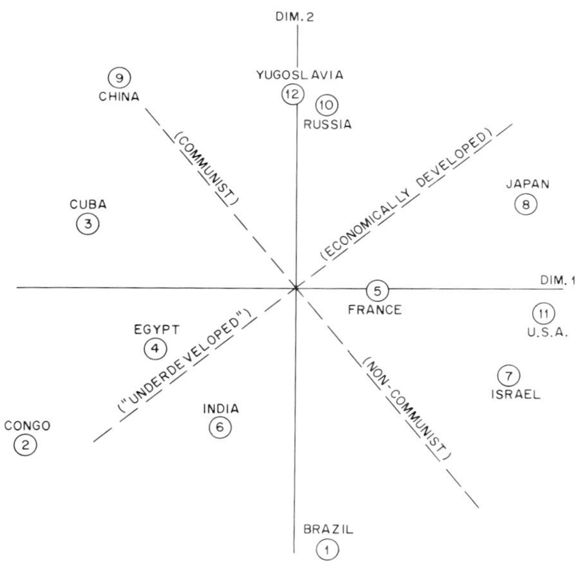

FIG. 6–*Two-dimensional solution from an M-D-SCAL analysis of averaged ratings of similarity among 12 nations (see Fig. 5). It was necessary to rotate the axes to interpret the dimensions.*

interpretation could be made of the third dimension of a three-dimensional M-D-SCAL solution.

Although these multidimensional results tell a great deal about the space for the average subject (since the matrix of averaged ratings was used as input), they provide no information about variations in the ways different people perceive nations. Until recently when data was available from several subjects or from the same subjects on different experimental occasions, one had only two options: (*a*) to do a single MDS of average proximities, treating the data from different individuals as experimental replications (as was done in the analysis just described); or (*b*) to do a separate scaling of each person's data, treating the data from different subjects as unrelated. There is now, however, another alternative, namely, to use Carroll and Chang's [*18*] INDSCAL (INdividual Differences SCALing) procedure. This new technique relates the spaces from different subjects in a strong way, while permitting large differences among them (see also Refs *19, 20,* and *21*).

Assumptions of the INDSCAL Model

The INDSCAL model shares with other MDS models the assumption that, for each individual, judgments of proximity are monotonically related to distance between stimuli in a multidimensional psychological space. However, each individual is assumed to have his (or her) own "private" perceptual space. A certain communality of perception is assumed, but this is balanced by the possibility of variation in the relative importance, or weight, of each dimension for different individuals. The INDSCAL model and method handles this notion of differential saliences of common dimensions by assuming that each individual's "private" space is derived from the common, or "group" stimulus space. (The group stimulus space corresponds to the multidimensional space obtained from M-D-SCAL or other earlier MDS procedures.) This is done by stretching or shrinking the dimensions of the group space in proportion to their perceptual importance for the particular individual.

The dimension weights for subjects can be plotted in another space, referred to as the "subject space." These weights can be interpreted as the squares of the stretching or shrinking factors for an individual. A stretching factor of zero means that the dimension has shrunk to the vanishing point—the individual attaches (consciously or unconsciously) no importance to the dimension; he does not perceive stimulus differences on that dimension or, in any case, acts as if he does not.

Besides providing a subject space, INDSCAL has another important advantage over the earlier MDS procedures; that is, it uses information in the individual differences (variation in subjects' proximities data) to orient the dimensions uniquely. Moreover, in most cases, the dimensions from INDSCAL can be interpreted without rotation of axes. As a result, it is generally much easier to interpret high-dimensional solutions from INDSCAL than from the earlier MDS procedures or factor analysis. (see Ref *15* for examples of five, six, and nine-dimensional INDSCAL solutions.)

An INDSCAL Analysis of the Nation Data

The INDSCAL procedure can be illustrated by a reanalysis of the data on perception of nations. In this case, the computer input was the set of 18 proximity matrices, one matrix per subject. The group stimulus space from a two-dimensional INDSCAL analysis is shown in Fig. 7*A*. As before, Dimensions 1 and 2 can be interpreted as "Political Alignment" (or Communist versus Noncommunist) and "Economic Development." (A three-dimensional analysis revealed another dimension which was interpreted as "Geography and Culture," since it distinguished the Western from the Eastern countries.) It was *not* necessary to rotate the axes to arrive at the interpretations since those arising from the INDSCAL analysis were directly interpretable.

The "subject space" from the INDSCAL analysis is shown in Fig. 7*B*. The *D, M,* or *H* in the circle representing a subject indicates whether the particular individual was classified as a "dove," "moderate," or "hawk" on the basis of supplementary information supplied by subjects in the questionnaire (concerning their views on the Vietnam war). One can see that there is a systematic relation between the relative importance of these dimensions and the subjects' political orientations. Thus, the "Political Alignment" dimension is more important for "hawks" than for "doves," while the "Economic Development" dimension is more important for "doves" than for "hawks."

The differences in perceptions of nations by "doves" and "hawks" is dramatized in Figs. 7*C* and 7*D,* which show Dimensions 1 and 2 of the "private" perceptual spaces for Subjects 17 (a "hawk") and 4 (a "dove"). The horizontal stretching of Subject 17's space reflects the fact that Dimension 1 is much more salient to him than Dimension 2. The vertical stretching of Subject 4's space is, likewise, the result of his higher weight on Dimension 2.

This example shows that INDSCAL can yield important information about both the stimuli and the individuals participating in the study. Moreover, the dimensions were easier to interpret than those from the M-D-SCAL analysis of the averaged data (Fig. 6) since no rotation was necessary.

Later studies[*15,16,22*] have revealed additional dimensions of nation perception. To show this, however, required a larger-scale study with more stimuli, subjects, and experimental tasks.

An INDSCAL Analysis of Helm's Color Vision Data

The remaining examples are in the area of visual perception. The data are from studies conducted by Helm[*23*] and by Indow and Kanazawa[*24*]. (We thank Professor Indow for supplying the raw data to us.)

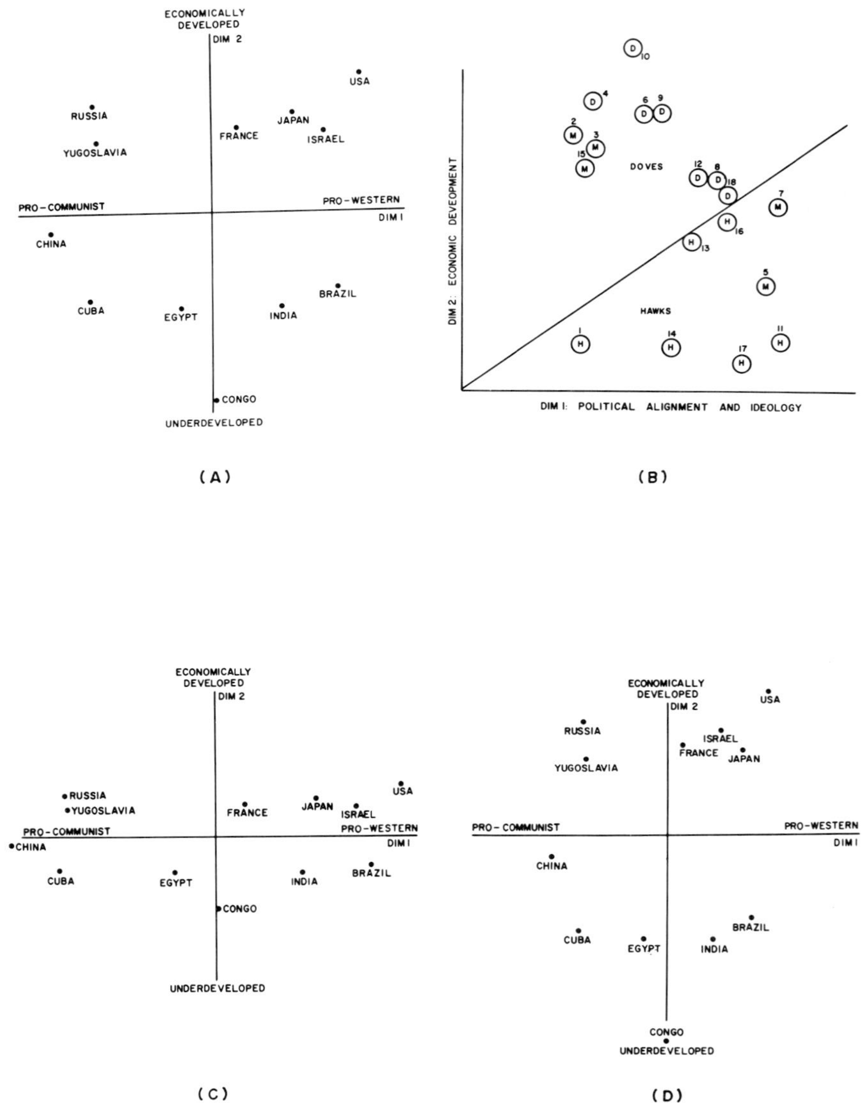

FIG. 7—*Dimensions 1 and 2 of* (A) *the group stimulus space and* (B) *the subject space from a two-dimensional INDSCAL analysis of 18 matrices of perceived similarities among nations*[16,17]. *The* D, M, *or* H *in a circle indicates whether the particular subject was classified as a "dove," "moderate," or "hawk" on the basis of his views on the Vietnam war. Figures* (C) *and* (D) *show the "private" perceptual spaces for subjects 17 and 4, respectively; these spaces were derived by applying the weights for these subjects* (*shown in* B) *to the dimensions of the group stimulus space* (*shown in* A).

The subjects in Helm's study judged psychological distances among ten colors of constant saturation and brightness. Their task was to arrange triples of color chips into triangles so that the length of the three sides were proportional to the perceived psychological distance between the color chips at the vertices. A matrix of psychological distances (the measure of proximity) was derived for each subject; in fact, there were two matrices apiece for two subjects who repeated the task on another occasion.

The entire set of matrices was used as input to INDSCAL[*15,25*]. The group stimulus space and the subject space, shown in Figs. 8 and 9, accounted for over 90 percent of the variance in the individual subjects' matrices. The space for the stimuli is the familiar color circle. Colors of constant saturation and brightness are represented on the circumference of a circle instead of on a straight line since, for example, violet and red (which are at opposite extremes of the visual portion of the electromagnetic spectrum) are more similar to each other psychologically than either is to green (which falls between violet and red on the spectrum). Again, the unrotated dimensions make sense; namely, there is a "red-green" and a "blue-yellow" dimension.

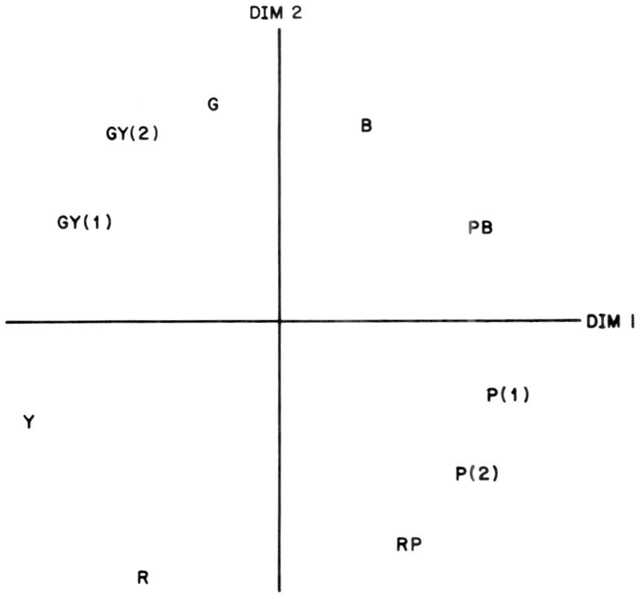

FIG. 8–*The group stimulus space from a two-dimensional INDSCAL analysis of Helm's*[23] *data on psychological distances among ten colors of constant saturation and brightness (see Ref* 25). *The coding of the colors is as follows:* R = *red;* Y = *yellow;* GY(1) = *green yellow;* GY(2) = *green yellow with more green than* GY(1); G = *green;* B = *blue;* PB = *purple blue;* P(1) = *purple;* P(2) = *purple with more red than* P(1); RP = *red purple.*

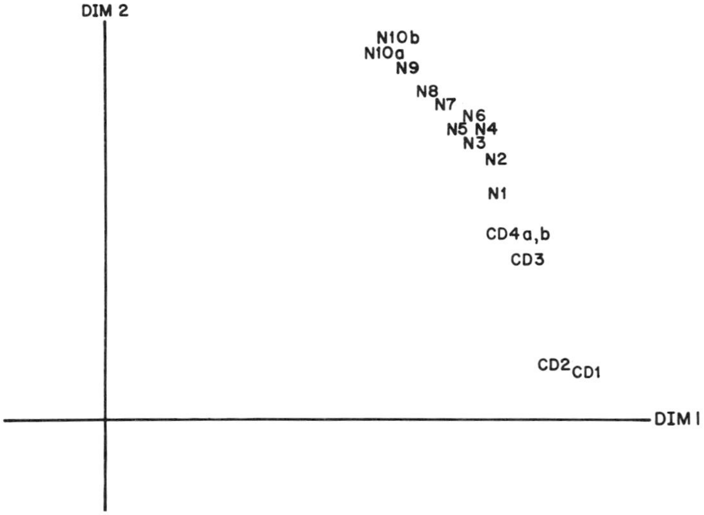

FIG. 9—*The subject space from a two-dimensional INDSCAL analysis of Helm's*[23] *data on psychological distances between ten colors of constant saturation and brightness. The N's correspond to subjects with normal color vision while the CD's are subjects with red-green color deficiencies.*

The subject space from the INDSCAL analysis, shown in Fig. 9, is quite illuminating. In this space CD1 through CD4 are four subjects with deficiencies in red-green color vision (CD4a and CD4b are two replications for the same subject), while N1 through N10 are ten subjects with normal color vision (N10a and N10b are replications). As would be predicted, all of the subjects with red-green color deficiences have lower weights on the red-green dimension than the "normal" subjects. Moreover, with one small reversal, the order of the weights for the four color-deficient subjects is consistent with the relative degree of deficiency, as reported by Helm. This suggests that the patterns of dimension weights from INDSCAL might be useful for diagnosing the degree of red-green color weakness, and perhaps also for diagnosing other deficiencies or anomalies in color vision. (Evidence for the usefulness of weights for diagnosing deficiencies in auditory perception is given in Ref *15.*)

The strength of the INDSCAL model and method is that it accommodates a wide range of perceptual variation in such a simple way. At the same time, it confirms in an elegant way what has been discovered by visual theorists using other procedures.

Perception of Colors Differing in Hue, Value, and Chroma

The final example of INDSCAL involves a reanalysis[*26*] of the Indow and Kanazawa[*24*] data on judged similarities of 24 colors varying in hue, value (brightness), and chroma (saturation). The four subjects who participated in the study made complete judgments via Indow's [*27*] method of multiple ratio judgments. The four resulting proximity matrices served as input to INDSCAL.

It should be kept in mind that in this, as well as in the preceding application, the knowledge about the dimensions of color perception was not "communicated to" the computer program. The program "saw" only the subjects' proximities data, and constructed the stimulus and subject spaces on the basis of this information alone.

Two planes of the "group" stimulus space for the Indow and Kanazawa data are shown in Figs. 10*A* and 10*B*. Dimensions 1 and 2 correspond reasonably well

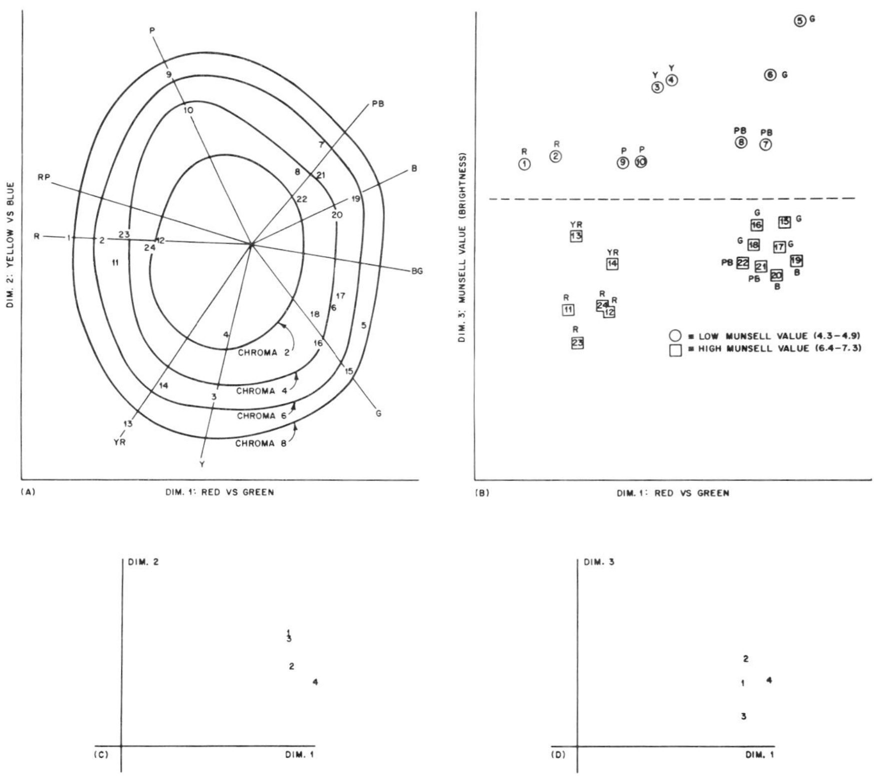

FIG. 10–*Planes of the group stimulus space,* (A) *and* (B), *and the subject space* (C) *and* (D), *from a three-dimensional INDSCAL analysis of the Indow and Kanazawa* [24] *data on similarities among colors differing in hue, value* (*brightness*) *and chroma* (*saturation*). *The "equichroma curves" and hue radii in* (A) *were drawn in by hand to clarify the interpretation of results. The coding of the colors in the group stimulus space is as follows:* R = *red;* RP = *red purple;* P = *purple;* PB = *purple blue;* B = *blue;* BG = *blue green;* G = *green;* Y = *yellow;* YR = *yellow red.*

to the "red-green" and "blue-yellow" dimensions. The concentric "circles" shown in Fig. 10*A* are "equichroma curves," ranging from Chroma 2 (inside) to Chroma 8 (outside). These curves and the hue radii were drawn in by hand solely to help the reader comprehend the figure. As shown in Fig. 10*B*, Dimension 3 reflects Munsell Value—all stimuli with low Munsell Value (4.3 to 4.9) are below the dashed line, while all with high Munsell Value (6.4 to 7.3) are above the line.

Indow and Kanazawa obtained a similar configuration for their data using an older MDS procedure to analyze the averaged proximities for the four subjects. However, they had to rotate the axes to find the structure we have displayed here. The uniqueness of orientation property of INDSCAL enabled us to find this interpretable structure without rotation. This is true despite the fact that there was negligible variation among subjects in weights for the dimensions. (Since INDSCAL relies on differences in patterns of subject weights to orient the axes, there is little guarantee of unique dimensions with such small differences in weights.) The lack of individual differences is shown in Figs. 10*C* and 10*D*, which plot the corresponding planes of the "subject space." The homogeneity of subjects resulted from Indow and Kanazawa's avoidance of subjects with deficient or anomalous color vision.

A study combining certain characteristics of the Helm and the Indow and Kanazawa studies would be very desirable—that is, color-deficient and anomalous subjects as well as subjects with normal color vision should be included, and the three-dimensional color space should be sampled as completely as possible. It is hard to predict just what the results would be since INDSCAL can find dimensions that are statistically related. Thus, it is conceivable that more than three dimensions would be required to account for the perceptions of all subjects, but with linear or nonlinear dependencies among them. An INDSCAL analysis of such data might shed light on these possibilities and increase our understanding of color perception.

Conclusions

Much that we have learned about the stimuli in these studies could have been learned by use of the older MDS methods, while other conclusions relied heavily on special properties of the newer INDSCAL procedure. To summarize, the major advantages of this new scaling technique are: (1) unique determination of dimensions, eliminating (in most cases) the need for rotation of coordinate axes to attain interpretability; (2) a parsimonious representation of data from many different perceptual "types" in a single and psychologically meaningful space; and (3) dimension weights for subjects which can be related to other variables of concern (for example, political orientation in the nation perception study, and color perception in the Helm study). INDSCAL, then, provides a very general method of quickly and efficiently learning a great deal about both the stimuli and the subjects under study, of confirming and improving on prior hypotheses about perception, and of graphically representing rather complex and subtle variations in multidimensional structures.

INDSCAL and the earlier MDS methods are of great practical as well as theoretical interest. MDS may not provide an instant solution to scientists' and engineers' research problems, but it can at least direct them to the variables most worthy of further study. The future holds promise of many new developments in the field of MDS and related techniques. There are new models to be explored, and new methods to be perfected and tried with real data. Yet it would seem that a strong start has been made and has already resulted in methods whose potential usefulness and range of applicability have only begun to be tapped.

References

[1] Shepard, R. N., *Psychometrika*, Vol. 27, 1962, pp. 125-140, 219-246.
[2] Shepard, R. N. in *Multidimensional Scaling: Theory and Applications in the Behavioral Sciences*, Vol. 1, *Theory*, R. N. Shepard, A. K. Romney, and S. Nerlove, Eds., Seminar Press, New York, 1972, pp. 21-47.
[3] Coombs, C. E., *A Theory of Data*, Wiley, New York, 1964.
[4] Torgerson, W. S., *Theory and Methods of Scaling*, Wiley, New York, 1958.
[5] Kruskal, J. B., *Psychometrika*, Vol. 29, 1964, pp. 1-27.
[6] Kruskal, J. B., *Psychometrika*, Vol. 29, 1964, pp. 115-129.
[7] Carroll, J. D. in *Multidimensional Scaling: Theory and Applications in the Behavioral Sciences*, Vol. 1, *Theory*, R. N. Shepard, A. K. Romney, and S. Nerlove, Eds., Seminar Press, New York, 1972, pp. 105-155.
[8] Wish, M., "Notes on the Variety, Appropriateness, and Choice of Proximity Measures," unpublished manuscript, Bell Laboratories, Murray Hill, N. J., 1972.
[9] Bricker, P. D., Johnson, S. C., and Mattke, C. F., *Behavioral Research Methods and Instrumentation*, Vol. 1, 1969, pp. 148-149.
[10] Pruzansky, S. "Judgments of Similarities Among Initial Consonants Using an Auditory Sorting Apparatus," presented at meetings of the Acoustical Society of America, Houston, Nov. 1970.
[11] Rosenberg, S., Nelson, C., and Vivekananthan, P. S., *Journal of Personality and Social Psychology*, Vol. 9, 1968, pp. 283-294.
[12] Wish, M., *Human Factors*, Vol. 9, 1967, pp. 529-539.
[13] Carroll, J. D. and Wish, M. in *Handbook of Perception*, Vol. 2, E. C. Carterette and M. P. Friedman, Eds., Academic Press, New York, 1974, in press.
[14] Miller, G. A. and Nicely, P. E., *Journal of the Acoustical Society of America*, Vol. 27, 1955, pp. 338-352.
[15] Wish, M. and Carroll, J. D. in *Handbook of Perception*, Vol. 2, E. C. Carterette and M. P. Friedman, Eds., Academic Press, New York, 1974, in press.
[16] Wish, M., Deutsch, M., and Biener, L., *Journal of Personality and Social Psychology*, Vol. 16, 1970, pp. 361-373.
[17] Wish, M. in *Attitude Research Reaches New Heights*, C. W. King and D. Tigert, Eds., American Marketing Association, Chicago, 1971, pp. 312-328.
[18] Carroll, J. D. and Chang, J. -J., *Psychometrika*, Vol. 35, 1970, pp. 283-319.
[19] Carroll, J. D. and Wish, M. in *Contemporary Developments in Mathematical Psychology*, Vol. 2, R. C. Atkinson, D. H. Krantz, R. D. Luce, and P. Suppes, Eds., W. H. Freeman, San Francisco, 1974, in press.
[20] Tucker, L. R. and Messick, S. J., *Psychometrika*, Vol. 28, 1963, pp. 333-367.
[21] Tucker, L. R., *Psychometrika*, Vol. 37, 1972, pp. 3-27.

[22] Wish, M. in *Proceedings,* 80th Annual Convention, American Psychological Association, 1972, pp. 301-302.
[23] Helm, C. E., *Journal of the Optical Society of America,* Vol. 54, 1964, pp. 256-262.
[24] Indow, T. and Kanazawa, K., *Journal of Experimental Psychology,* Vol. 59, 1960, pp. 330-336.
[25] Carroll, J. D. and Chang, J. -J. in *Proceedings,* 78th Annual Convention, American Psychological Association, 1970, pp. 137-138.
[26] Carroll, J. D. "Multidimensional Scaling of Visual Stimuli," presented at meetings of the Optical Society of America, Ottawa, Oct. 1971.
[27] Indow, T. in *Handbook of Perception,* Vol. 2, E. C. Carterette and M. P. Friedman, Eds., Academic Press, New York, 1973, in press.

A. C. Little[1]

Color Evaluation of Foods—Correlation of Objective Facts with Subjective Impressions

REFERENCE: Little, A. C., "**Color Evaluation of Foods–Correlation of Objective Facts with Subjective Impressions,**" *Sensory Evaluation of Appearance of Materials, ASTM STP 545,* American Society for Testing and Materials, 1973, pp. 109-127.

ABSTRACT: In the early 1950's, a symposium entitled Color in Foods was arranged under the aegis of the National Academy of Sciences, National Research Council. The proceedings of that symposium have not to this day been superseded by a more up-to-date consideration of the state of knowledge as it has evolved since then.

At that time, considerable discussion was focused on the question of the validity of relating objective data to some visually determined and presumably imprecise scale. Because the opportunity has not presented itself to continue the vigorous exploration of this and other unresolved questions, the reservations and recommendations expressed in the proceedings stand unchallenged.

It is the purpose of this report to present a detailed discussion of the procedural framework developed by us to provide the basis for developing solutions for specific commodities and for specific purposes. The essentials include the development of model systems constructed to vary in known and controlled fashion along the requisite dimensions of color; the determination of optimum conditions for analyzing samples precisely and reproducibly for changes in physical and chemical properties which underlie changes in perceived color; the definition and construction of psychological scales which provide data relevant to the case in point; and finally, the demonstration of a highly significant relationship between visual evaluations and physically determined quantities. Thus, for different products, the same conceptual model is used; yet the procedural details may differ widely depending on the constraints imposed by physical and chemical characteristics of the sample and the specific requirements of the case. The feasibility of the approach will be explored with reference to actual examples.

KEY WORDS: senses, perception, color, colorimetry, visual perception

The year 1931 marked an event of historical significance after 200 years of observations, investigations, and theorizing on the physics, psychology, and

[1] Associate food scientist and lecturer, University of California, Dept. of Nutritional Sciences, Berkeley, Calif. 94720.

psychophysics of light, color, and vision starting with Newton in the early 18th century and including Young, Grassmann, von Helmholtz, and Maxwell in the 19th century, and later in the 20th century with Guild, Wright, and august members of the Optical Society of America on Colorimetry. Reference is made, of course, to the Standard Observer and Coordinate System recommended by the International Commission on Illumination (CIE)[*1*] [2] which has provided the basis for the ever-expanding science and technology of colorimetry. Coincident with the definition of the CIE system was the development by Hardy at the Massachusetts Institute of Technology of the first recording spectrophotometer for measuring reflectance and transmittance characteristics. The original instrument described in 1929[*2*] was designed for 0, 45 deg illumination and viewing, but this was almost immediately superseded by the prototype with integrating sphere built at MIT in 1935, the direct ancestor of the present day General Electric Recording Spectrophotometer[*3*].

The following year, Hardy's monumental *Handbook of Colorimetry* [*4*] was published by the MIT Press, thus making available the means of reducing spectrophotometric data to colorimetric specifications incorporating standard sources A, B, or C, at wavelength intervals as small as 1 nm if desired, covering range from 380 to 770 nm. The stage was thus set for the rapid proliferation of instrumentation for and application of what is frequently referred to as the "objective measurement of color." Transformation of the irregular spacing of just-noticeable-difference steps on the CIE-chromaticity diagram to uniform chromaticity diagrams were soon proposed ([*5*] pp. 290-300 and [*6*] Chapter 7) to provide single-number evaluations of color differences among samples.

As early as 1937, reports began to appear describing the development of broad-band filter photometers for the direct measurement of tri-stimulus values of opaque samples, followed in 1948 by the first-generation Hunter Color and Color Difference Meter, providing data in Hunter *L, a, b* space[*7*]. The ostensibly uniform lightness and chromaticness spacing provided the basis for calculating color differences, ΔE, in Euclidean geometry by determining the hypoteneuse of the right-triangle formed by connecting the distance ΔL (the lightness difference) with the distance $[(\Delta a)^2 + (\Delta b)^2]^{1/2}$ thus:

$$\Delta E = [(\Delta L)^2 + (\Delta a)^2 + (\Delta b)^2]^{1/2}$$

The directness and simplicity of measurement and computation by the Hunter approach soon led to wide acceptance which continues to this day.

Particular mention is made here to instrumentation yielding results in Hunter space because of the prevalence of application to problems of color evaluation of foods. The catalog of instruments is extensive, including both spectrophotom-

[2] The italic numbers in brackets refer to the list of references appended to this paper.

eters and colorimeters with various geometries of illumination and viewing of greater or lesser sophistication so far as data processing is concerned, ranging widely in precision and reproducibility, designed for diverse purposes as a research tool with demanding performance characteristics on one extreme to a rugged control instrument for field use on the other extreme.

The CIE system does not properly qualify as a method for the objective color measurement; in fact, it is precisely a color-stimulus specification expressed in terms of stimulus equivalents. Thus, the three-number specification, the XYZ tristimulus values, or, more often, the Y tristimulus value and the x and y chromaticity coordinates, simply identifies the composition of the additive mixture of the CIE primaries which will exactly match visually, but not necessarily spectrally, the sample in question when viewed by the 2 deg Standard Observer under defined conditions of illumination and viewing. Such data provide a permanent record, eschew the need for material standards, and can easily be incorporated into computer programs and storage and retrieval systems. No great stretch of the imagination is needed to appreciate the remarkable versatility of such an internationally recognized psychophysical system.

Applications of Colorimetry

Applications of colorimetry can be conveniently divided into two categories: (1) in the manufacture of materials to specification and (2) in the characterization of objects as they exist. In the former case, the CIE specification can be considered, to all intents and purposes, to constitute a color requirement (that is, it defines the requisite color stimulus). Here, specifications are written to ensure that the color or color reproduction ability of the manufactured item will conform to predetermined criteria, with emphasis placed on matching a designated counterpart, within defined tolerance limits. The list of applications falling in this category is virtually endless; paints, dyes and chemical coatings, ceramics, glass, plastics, textiles, paper, building materials, code and signal displays, printing, photography, and color television to name some of the obvious and prevalent ones.

The latter category includes all naturally occurring animal, vegetable, and mineral matter where interest is focused on identification, classification, and description of attributes visually perceived as color. Here, colorimetry should be viewed as an analytical tool from which information can be extracted pertaining to chemical and physical characteristics of the object identifiable as the physical correlates to visual color experience. This point will be explored in greater detail with reference to foods.

Foods as examples of naturally occurring biological materials occupy a position of particular importance in this category because visual appearance plays an important role in consumer acceptability and is an important indicator of quality at all stages from selection of raw materials to recognition of early deterioration on storage. Colorimetric analysis thus provides information regarding the conditions of a food as it exists at a given time.

Any naturally occurring object can be characterized and classified in similar fashion, and indeed examples are numerous. Apart from foods, agricultural products such as cotton, tobacco, and wool have a long history of colorimetric evaluation. Studies continue on structural colors in many animals and even a few plants [*8,9*] as well as on colors generated from the presence of natural pigments.

Problems in astronomy, meterology, and underwater visibility provide examples of the use of colorimetry in establishing the relationship of physical information with visual experience.

Interestingly, a very early publication [*10*], predating by one year the 1931 CIE *Proceedings* [*1*], concerns analysis of colors produced in structures under strain in photoelastic experiments by the tristimulus system.

Interest in the application of colorimetry of reflecting surfaces to foods developed rapidly among food scientists and technologists, with a report on spectrophotometric and colorimetric analyses of tomato pulp published in 1937 [*11*]. Following the restrictions imposed by World War II, reports began appearing in the literature in 1946 from Kramer's laboratory at the University of Maryland, followed in rapid succession by publications from other academic institutions; notably, the Universities of California, Massachusetts, Oregon State, and Purdue; USDA laboratories, industry, and the Quartermaster Food and Container Institute. This early activity culminated in a two day symposium on color in foods in November 1953, sponsored by the Quartermaster Food and Container Institute for the Armed Forces and the National Academy of Science, National Research Council. Particular reference is made to the *Proceedings* published the following year [*12*] despite the fact that no reference sources listed there are now less than 20 years old. It might therefore be argued that developments over the past two decades have rendered the publication obsolete. The symposium, however, represents a unique event, never repeated since to the same degree of participation with the consequent opportunity for a free exchange of ideas and opinions by investigators interested in colorimetry of foods. Therefore, the impact exerted by the *Proceedings* continues to manifest itself to this day. That is not to say that activity in this area has died out nor that there has been a lack of publications and presentations at meetings during the intervening years. The point is that the opportunity to reevaluate the points of view expressed in the *Proceedings* and to examine critically recent developments in an open forum has not presented itself.

While this report cannot and does not purport to provide that opportunity, its purpose is to present a personal statement of our concept of colorimetry as it applies to foods, with specific examples to illustrate the adaptation of the general concept to fit the requirements of a particular case. A review of current literature is not intended; literature references are cited in the main only when applicable to the development of the discussion.

A General Approach to Color Evaluation of Foods

Color Evaluation of Foods–A Distinct Category

As suggested earlier, the major rationale for the development of the CIE Standard Observer, Standard Coordinate System, and its subsequent transformations to systems with perceptually uniform spacings (or a reasonable facsimile) was to provide an unambiguous method of reducing spectrophotometric data to stimulus equivalents specifications under defined conditions of illumination and viewing for objects manufactured to color requirements. The indisputable value of such data lies in their ability to predict the conditions for attaining visual matches between spectrally dissimilar objects, the so-called "metameric" or "conditional" matches generated by invisible spectral differences. Color tolerances define the limits of differences that will still result in acceptable matches, and changes in colorimetric values with time can yield information regarding colorfastness, fading, soiling, etc. The present and potential applications of stimulus equivalents specifications are vast, yet one is hard pressed to think of a single example where metameric matching is of concern in the manufacture of foods, and few where an exact spectral match is demanded. When the color of a food is developed by the addition of colorants, through blending of ingredients, or through processing to a desired color end point, the objective is to obtain not exact matches but acceptable colors that do not differ unduly from batch to batch. The consumer accepts reasonable consistency in the color of roasted coffee but demands exact matches in the ceramic tiles in the shower stall.

The essential difference between the consideration of the color of a food and that of a manufactured item, that is, the evaluation of the color of the former as it exists at a given time in contrast to the controlled combination of ingredients to yield a product with a designated colorimetric specification, provides the basis for the argument presented here that the tools and techniques applicable to one category may not be and often are not transferable to the other.

A further point to be made regarding the differences in purpose for evaluating color in foods and in manufactured items is that with foods, color is a reflection of state or condition at a given time, it therefore can be used as a criterion for grading or ranking in terms of monetary value, quality, or acceptability. While product rejection can occur, for example, in raw material selection or termination of shelflife, it is frequently not a question of yes or no, but A, B, or C grade. With products manufactured to a given color requirement, the question is one of accept or reject, for which tolerance limits are defined. Here, interest is focused on color *per se.*

Despite the wide diversity in physical form which exists among the items covered by the generic term "food," there are certain common properties which provide the impetus for developing a model for color evaluation of foods which can be adapted to the particular characteristics, constraints, and requirements imposed by a specific commodity.

In general, the perceived color of a food owes its origin to the presence of naturally occurring pigment systems in various combinations and concentrations, distributed in diverse fashion throughout the structure of the food and to the physical structure of the food. Foods can be opaque solids of various degrees of pigmentation covering a wide range in size and shape, whole or subdivided; semisolid translucent gels and purées which absorb and scatter incident light, turbid liquids, pigmented or not; clear liquids, essentially non-scattering, but containing various concentrations of pigments with specific light-absorbing properties.

Changes in light-modifying properties and, thus, the perceived color of foods can be due to factors such as changes in pigment composition with growth and maturation of the plant or animal, exposure to radiant energy, changes in pH, changes in the redox, variation in particle size, addition of fats or oils, browning or scorching, and modification of cellular structure. It is immediately recognized that the factors responsible for the genesis and modification of color also determine the physical and chemical state and properties of components of the system, and thus, the measure of one can be used to predict the measure of the other. It is the realization of these interrelationships that has caused us to question the general applicability of stimulus equivalents specifications to color evaluations of foods, particularly specifications based on uniform color spaces, for example, L, a, b, or U^*, V^*, W^*.

While the CIE XYZ or Y, x, y values do provide information regarding the spectral transmittance or reflectance properties as measured by three broad band filters, nothing is gained by the incorporation of a standard source, and, in fact, the information pertaining to the relative contributions in the red and the blue may be distorted by incorporating the small blue hump in the calculation of X and by arbitrarily adjusting the magnitude of the blue. When data are presented in terms of L, a, b or U^*, V^*, W^* or some other transformation of X, Y, and Z, the description of the stimulus in terms of its equivalent or match has completely superseded the description of the stimulus in terms of its light-modifying properties. It should be abundantly apparent by now that with foods, the latter is of far greater interest than the former. The calculation of ΔE, the color differences among samples by any one of several methods merely gives an estimate of perceptibility difference steps without indicating the parameters involved or the direction of differences.

The Proposed Model for Color Evaluation of Foods

The basic model for exploring the interrelationship of the light-modifying properties of foods, (and by extension, biological systems in general) to visual color perception and to chemical and physical properties of the system is as follows:

1. the object,
2. the synthetic process,
3. the analytical process, and
4. the analytical process as a predictor of the synthetic process.

The Object—The object (the sample), on which our interest is focused, may be opaque, translucent, or transparent with properties of absorbing, reflecting, transmitting, and scattering incident light. Pigment distribution can range from a single homogenously distributed pigment system to a random distributed multicomponent system. The degree of complexity is a major factor in determining the conditions of sample preparation for presentation to the instrument.

Synthetic Process—The synthetic process is effected by the observer who by virtue of the retinal receptor system, optic nerve, cerebral cortex complex translates the qualitative and quantitative distribution of light activating the receptor system to visual color perception. Observer judgments are evaluated by psychological scaling techniques, among which ranking, rating, and paired comparisons have provided useful information. Independent information regarding color vision and color discrimination ability is obtained from screening tests, the HRR-PIC and the Ishihara Plate Tests, and color discrimination and color aptitude testing procedures, notably, the F-M 100 Hue Test and the ISCC-CAT, currently being evaluated for effectiveness in predicting the ability of observers to make required visual judgments [*13,14*].

Analytical Process—The analytical process involves the determination of spectral reflectance or transmittance characteristics or both of the sample as prepared for precise, reproducible analysis [*15-17*]. A successful resolution of the problem of defining the analytical procedure is facilitated by independent knowledge of the chemical composition and physical characteristics of the system, obtained through construction of model systems or by alternative analytical procedures. In turn, the determination of reflectance or transmittance characteristics can be used to deduce certain chemical and physical properties of the system. Model systems may be prepared by combining materials of known properties in various combinations to simulate a food; by the addition of controlled increments of pigment to a food; by blending two components by systematically changing the composition of the mixture; by controlled oxidative degradation of a pigment system; by addition of light scattering particles to a non-turbid medium etc.

Analytical Process as a Predictor of the Synthetic Process—This is defined through the determination of a highly significant relationship between objectively determined quantities and visual evaluations, namely, the psychophysical relationship. The objectively determined quantities can range from reflectance or transmittance measurements across the visible spectrum reduced to *XYZ* or *RGB,* to isolated portions of the light stimulus such as single or weighted combinations of broad or narrow-band measurements, to levels of nonvisible components. The latter is particularly useful in the instances where changes in the levels of ultraviolet absorbing components can be shown to parallel exactly the development of color through the nonenzymatic browning reaction as demonstrated with roasting of coffee [*18*].

Just as it is important to gain information regarding the performance characteristics of the human eye when used as an instrument to make critical color judgments, so too must the performance characteristics of the spectrophotometer or colorimeter be known. Methods of calibrating instruments to yield comparable data must be defined for any method to be proposed for general application. One approach involves establishing linear relationships between a designated "standard" instrument and test instruments ([*6*] p. 245).

The concept of the basic model, as just presented, was developed from observations made during the course of study of a number of transparent, translucent, and opaque systems. While the need to standardize rigorously the conditions of sample preparation and presentation to the instrument for evaluation of color had long been recognized, the extension of the techniques of colorimetry to the analysis of chemical components and optical properties has gradually evolved only relatively recently. The groundwork for this development is to be found in a report on the measurement of color of translucent samples [*19*]. In the course of attempting to measure reflectance characteristics of a series of samples of apple sauce to which had been added successive increments of raspberry purée by what were at that time considered acceptable techniques, it was noted that the reflectometer was not capable of ranking the samples in order of increasing redness, that is, increasing concentration of anthocyanin pigment, a task which was competently performed by the visual panelists.

A method was evolved involving measurement of thin layers of sample, backed alternately with a white, highly reflecting surface and a black, almost totally light absorbing surface. By application of Kubelka-Munk analysis, ([*5*] p. 395) it is possible to evaluate the internal transmittance, T_i, absorption and scattering coefficients, K and S, respectively; and reflectivity of infinite depth, R_∞, calculated from three measurements for each of the three values: R, R_o, and R_g. R is the reflectance of layer with white background (of reflectance R_g); R_o is the reflectance of layer with black background; and R_g is the reflectance of white background on which sample is placed. R_∞ is the difference between two quantities a and b, where

$$a = \frac{(S+K)}{S} = 1/2 \left[R + \frac{(R_O - R + R_g)}{R_O R_g} \right]$$

and

$$b = (a^2 - 1)^{1/2}$$

From the foregoing:

$$K = S(a - 1)$$

and S is derived from the expression:

$$SX = \frac{1}{b} \text{Ar ctgh} \frac{(1 - aR_O)}{bR_O}$$

For the general expressions involving R, the corresponding X, Y, and Z values are substituted to obtain the optical characteristics of the sample in the "red," "green," and "blue" regions of the spectrum as measured with three broad band filters with spectral distributions approximating those of the color-mixing functions of the standard observer, $\bar{x}$, $\bar{y}$, and $\bar{z}$, as proposed by Little[*19*].

The values obtained from the thin-layer white-background measurements were found to separate the samples with a high degree of sensitivity with changes in the chromaticity coordinates x and y completely in accord with the controlled changes in pigment concentration and more precisely than visual judgments. Similar results were obtained with a model system consisting of agar, cellulose fiber, and systematic increments of beta-carotene. It was concluded that direct measurement of the surface reflectance characteristics of such translucent, light-scattering samples failed to separate them in proper order because the photocell could not distinguish between light lost by selective absorption from light lost by internal transmission and scattering and the application of thin-layer methodology avoided this confusion. As color perception is a synthetic process, the observer is not limited in this way.

Application of the Model to Specific Examples

To illustrate how, in practice, the model just presented applies to specific examples of foods and beverages, a brief resumé is now presented for a few commodities which have been studied in our laboratory, touching only on the salient features with a summary presented in Table 1. Detailed descriptions of most of the studies have already appeared in the literature.

TABLE 1—*Summary of the model applied to five foods and beverages with various physical and chemical properties.*

Example	The Sample	Synthetic Process	Analytical Process	Analytical Process as Predictor of Synthetic Process
(1) Canned Tuna	Opaque, irregularly pigmented with labile pigment system. High specific absorption.	10 point scale, very light (10) to very dark (1).	Reflectance measurements under oxidizing and reducing conditions	(*a*) Highly significant relationship between *Y* (or *G*) value scale and visual point scale (p = 0.001). (*b*) Magnitude of chromaticity shift related to relative concentration of pigment.
(2) Applesauce	Translucent, moderately light-scattering, low absorption.	Rank order of samples prepared to vary in browning (illumination critical for accurate ranking).	Thin-layer transreflectometry, calculation of Kubelka-Munk optical constants.	Unidimensional scales $-\log T_{iZ}$ and Z_∞ both give precise measure of browning of applesauce in line with visual ranking.
(3) Milk	Highly turbid, moderately light transmitting. Low absorption.	Rank order of samples with increasing butterfat content (a very difficult task).	Thin-layer transreflectometry, calculation of Kubelka-Munk optical constants.	$-\text{Log}\ T_{iX}$ and $-\log T_{iY}$ yield precise measures o of increasing butterfat content, analytical process sensitive without error, synthetic, high incidence of error.
(4) White Wine	Highly transparent, very low to no turbidity, very low absorption.	Rank order of samples prepared to correspond to 0.1 to 1.0 Lovibond at intervals of 0.05 Lovibond.	Thin-layer transreflectometry or newly designed White Wine Colorimeter.	Perfect relationship among $-\log Z$ or *B*, Lovibond equivalent, and visual ranking.
(5) Red and Rosé Wines	Moderate to low transmittance, moderate to high absorption, very low turbidity.	Rank order of blends of red and white, red and rosé, etc.	Thin-layer transreflectometry.	Three dimensional diagram— $-\log X$ or *R*, $-\log Y$ or *G* $-\log Z$ or *B* for describing and predicting color of blends.

Example 1–An Opaque, Light-Diffusing System with Well-Defined Absorption Maxima–Canned Tuna [20]–The objective of this study was to develop an instrumental method for classifying the color of canned tuna to replace the Federal Standard of Identity definition based on a visual comparison with Munsell neutral value papers. The cut-off points for white, light and dark samples were thus already established in terms of Munsell V which is easily translated to CIE Y value according to the relationship defined by the Optical Society of America ([5] p. 430, [6] Appendix C).

The sample–Canned tuna consists of muscle fiber irregularly pigmented with a denatured globin hemochrome, usually processed in an oil medium. On opening the can, particularly of the white or light meat packs, the muscle fibers are seen to be streaked a delicate pink color which fades rapidly on exposure to air, thus indicating the extreme lability of the pigment in the presence of oxygen. The concentration of pigment determines in large part the reflectance level and thus the classification white, light or dark. As prepared for instrument presentation, the sample is opaque, light diffusing with specific absorptive properties.

To establish observer sensitivity to small steps in color difference, it should be possible to prepare a series of samples varying in small controlled difference steps by sequential addition of dark to light samples. Because we were interested in comparing panel score ratings with measured values, a statistical approach was used.

The synthetic process–Samples were evaluated on a ten point scale from 10 (very light) to 1 (very dark) by a trained panel. Unusual or off-color appearance was identified by qualifying terms; tan, very red, and very brown.

The analytical process–A method was evolved for obtaining precise, reproducible reflectance measurements with tristimulus colorimeters for samples exposed to atmospheric oxygen and under reducing conditions. The magnitude of the shift in chromaticity coordinates x and y on reduction of the air oxidized sample with sodium dithionite yielded a relative measure of intact denatured globin hemochrome. Spectral reflectance curves for a sample prepared under oxidizing and reducing conditions are shown in Fig. 1. Changes in the reversibility and magnitude of the shift on exposure of samples to oxidizing conditions for long periods of time led to the postulation of a two-stage sequence of events to describe the oxidative degradation, with the first stage rapid and reversible; the second, slow and irreversible. Antioxidants inhibited deterioration by blocking the reaction sequence at the first stage, suggesting that they inhibit rupture of the heme ring.

The feasibility of proposing the method for industry wide use, and for inclusion in standard definitions was explored, with the result that plastic standards were produced to enable calibration of instruments to conform to a designated standard instrument.

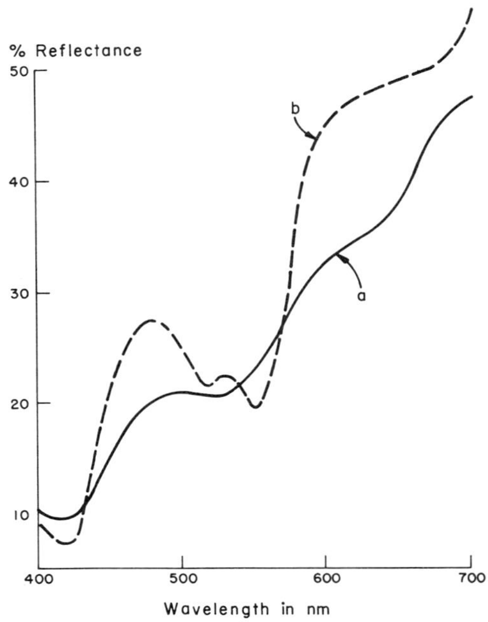

FIG. 1–*Reflectance spectra of canned tuna:* (a) *Pigment in the oxidized or ferri-hemochrome state,* (b) *Pigment in the reduced or ferro-hemochrome state. The chromaticity shift provides a measure of the difference between two curves.*

During the course of the investigation, numerous spectrophotometric reflectance spectra were obtained to follow changes in absorption characteristics following various experimental manipulations. Certain observations of the character and detail of the curves obtained after sample exposure to oxidizing and to reducing conditions provided insights into the interplay of light absorption by the pigment and light-scattering by the essentially neutral cellular matrix with which the pigment is associated. The ratio of the scattering coefficient S_λ to the absorption coefficient K_λ appears to be the critical relationship. With S_λ/K_λ large, the scattering effect may mask the pigment effect. As K_λ increases, the ratio decreases, and the masking effect is reduced.

A recent publication by Clydesdale [*17*] reiterates the potential importance of this relationship in the production of food products designed with consumer acceptability and nutritive value in mind.

The analytical process as a predictor of the synthetic process–A highly significant relationship was found to exist between the level of reflectance expressed as Y value (green reflectance) of the air-exposed samples and visual scores ($p = 0.001$). Because the red and blue reflectance values paralleled the green, their inclusion in the regression analysis did not significantly affect the relationship.

The measurement of chromaticity shift on reduction with sodium dithionite proved a valuable adjunct to the direct reflectance measurements where measured values and visual scores were not in accord. In such samples, the reflectance value is dependent only in part on pigment content, but also to degradative oxidation, scorching, or browning.

Example 2–A Translucent Light Scattering Purée with Poorly Defined Absorption Characteristics–Applesauce [13]–The problem was to explore the possibility of using thin-layer transreflectometry for purposes of evaluating visual attributes and calculating optical constants based on Kubelka-Munk theory for a highly translucent, virtually nonpigmented system.

The sample–Applesauce was selected as fulfilling the stated requirements. It is a nonstructured semisolid with low absorption characteristics. Samples differing in controlled fashion were prepared by the addition of small increments of caramelized applesauce to the non-browned starting product.

The synthetic process–Observers selected for good color discrimination ability were given the task of rank ordering samples prepared to differ sequentially by small intervals. The observers performed the experiment under two light sources, one simulating standard Source A (2854°K) and the second, standard Source C (6740°K). Samples were evaluated with greater accuracy under Source C than Source A.

The analytical process–Red, green, and blue transreflectometric values were obtained for samples in glass cells backed by white and by black reflecting surfaces, respectively. From the measured quantities, optical constants were calculated: T_1, the internal transmittance; R_∞, the reflectivity of an infinite depth; K, the absorption coefficient; and S, the scattering coefficient.

The analytical process as a predictor of the synthetic process–The reciprocal log function of internal transmittance and R_∞ for the Z value (blue transreflectance) provided the most sensitive means of evaluating sample differences and, thus, either value could provide the basis for psychophysical scales in this case.

The amount of browning that a product of this kind has undergone on storage can thus be estimated by the appropriate –log function.

Example 3–A Turbid Liquid with Low Light Absorption Properties–Homogenized Milk [13]–The objective of this experiment was to find a suitable method of measuring differences among samples varying in butter fat content and to observe how these differences affect appearance.

The sample–Milk is a very turbid liquid of complex composition. It is moderately translucent with low light absorption properties. A series of samples was prepared by addition of measured increments of whole milk to fat free milk.

The synthetic process–Visual panelists were asked to rank samples according to increasing turbidity or "milkiness" under artificial daylight (Source C) illumination. This proved a difficult task with less than 60 percent correct judgments.

The analytical process—Thin-layer transreflectometric readings with white and black backgrounds were obtained, and the optical constants were calculated as previously described. The $-\log T_i$ for both the X and Y values proved equally sensitive indicators of differences in sample composition, yielding parallel linear relationships as shown in Fig. 2.

The analytical process as a predictor of the synthetic process—This case represents a situation where an instrumental method far exceeds the human eye in ability to distinguish differences among samples.

Example 4—A Highly Transparent, Essentially Nonturbid, Low-Absorbing Liquid—White Wine [21]—The objective of this study was to develop a precise, reproducible method of evaluating white wine color to conform to the rigorous Federal Specification which limits the color of white wines to a designation described as "no less than 0.6 Lovibond in a 1/2 inch cell." The official method involves measurement of absorption at 430 nm with a monochromator that meets certain design and performance criteria. This method has been found inadequate in practice, and, therefore, an alternative procedure was sought.

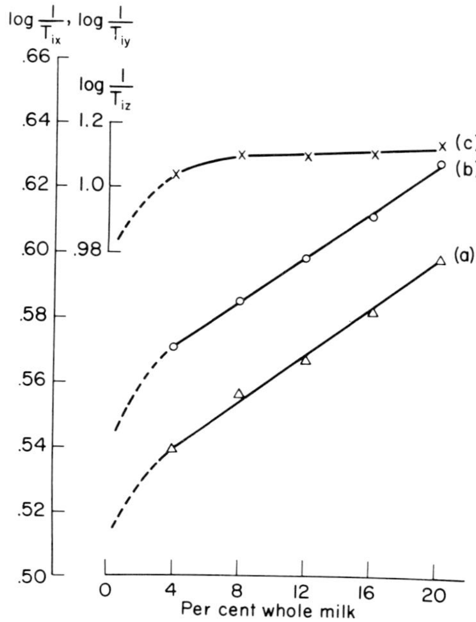

FIG. 2—*Addition of whole milk to skim milk:* (a) $-\log T_{iX}$ (b) $-\log T_{iY}$ (c) $-\log T_{iZ}$

The sample—White wines that approach the 0.6 Lovibond requirement are virtually water white when viewed in a test tube or ordinary wine glass. Wines of increasing Lovibond number are increasingly yellow in color. A bottled finished white wine is essentially nonturbid. To provide a series of samples of light white wines differing sequentially in small steps, the starting material was diluted with 12 percent alcohol or blended with a darker white wine.

The synthetic process—Panelists were asked to rank white wines in test tubes held against a white backing and illuminated by front lighting with an incandescent lamp and diffuse overhead artificial daylight. Very small differences were perceived with a high degree of accuracy of the order of 0.05 Lovibond corresponding to a difference in A_{430} of about 0.004 in a 1 cm cell.

The analytical process—The direct measurement of the blue or Z transreflectometric value of white wine samples in a glass cell backed with a white reflecting standard proved far superior to the spectrophotometric method as defined by the Association of Official Analytical Chemists [*22*]. Where the spectrophotometric method could not distinguish samples differing to the order of 0.05 Lovibond, a critical difference in the legal requirement, the transreflectometric method successfully resolved even smaller intervals without error. A major source of error proved to be attributable to subliminal turbidity, not visible to the eye, but affecting grossly the A_{430} reading, predictable from Raleigh's equation which states that scatter is inversely proportional to the fourth power of wavelength. For solutions with low specific absorption, this becomes intolerable. The subliminal turbidity effect was proven by measuring absorption at 430 and 750 nm (which should be 0 for nonturbid samples) with a directional and a sphere spectrophotometer. The latter gives a measure of total transmittance, directional plus scatter, and the difference between the two measurements at 430 nm is thus a measure of the contribution of the Raleigh scattering.

These findings led to the design and construction of a new transmittance meter, the White Wine Colorimeter, to implement the principles of the transreflectometric technique ([*21*] p. 203). The source, filter, sample, and detector are placed in close juxtaposition resembling an "extended sandwich." The diameter of the receptor is equal to the diameter of the sample cell, and thus forward scattered light is included, and the subliminal turbidity effect no longer is a problem. The instrument has been thoroughly tested in the laboratory and in the field with complete success.

The analytical process as a predictor of the synthetic process—This is a case where an exact relationship can be found between the objective method and visual evaluation, provided that the constraints imposed by the optical properties of the instrument and the sample are taken into consideration and that visual evaluations are made under optimal conditions of illumination and viewing, by observers with good visual discrimination. The directional spectrophotometer could not do the job, because the photocell could not distinguish between light lost due to absorption from light lost due to scatter. The visual process does not suffer from this handicap.

White wines owe their color to polymerization products of ultraviolet absorbing components which causes a shift in absorption maximum to the short wavelength region of the visible spectrum. Therefore, the unidimensional scale completely evaluates the color as well as the extent of nonenzymatic browning which has taken place.

Example 5–Light Transmitting, Essentially Nonturbid Liquids with Moderate to High Specific Absorption–Red and Rosé Wines [23]–In this case, the objective was to develop a method of blending red and rosé wines to specific color requirements, using transreflectometric measurements as the basis for determining the blend composition.

The sample–Red and rosé wines are more or less pigmented with anthocyanins and can also contain various amounts of products of the browning reaction. Anthocyanins also act as indicators by changing color with pH. Red and rosé wines are thus far more complex in composition than white wines, at least so far as the components giving rise to color are concerned.

The synthetic process–Visual evaluations involved ranking wines prepared to differ by small steps as previously described, and comparing samples blended to meet a color requirement according to the method described later with a sample of the target color. The illuminating and viewing conditions become increasingly critical as the wines being evaluated become more heavily pigmented. Even under the most favorable conditions, panelists experienced increasing difficulty in discriminating differences with increasing pigmentation.

The analytical process–The thin-layer transreflectometric technique was successfully adapted to the complete range of wine colors by varying cell depth to provide optimal resolution of wines falling within certain ranges, namely, white, amber, rosé, medium red, and dark red. Blends were made by combining different starting wines (some already blended from a number of wines) to form series varying in known, controlled fashion. When the –log of the *R, G,* and *B* or *X, Y,* and *Z* transreflectometric readings of samples backed with a white reflecting surface were plotted against composition of the blend, curvilinear relationships were obtained with an essentially linear relationship pertaining at moderate to low absorption values. The slopes of the three linear portions differ according to spectral region, with the steepest slope for the –log *B*. With two starting wines, a graph can be constructed which shows the relationship of red to green to blue or *X* to *Y* to *Z* transreflectance for any mixture of the two wines. An example of the sequential blending of a white and a rosé is shown in Fig. 3. Given two starting wines and a color requirement, the composition of the required blend can be read from the chart directly. The percent composition scale is adjustable within the limits of the extremes so that final adjustments can

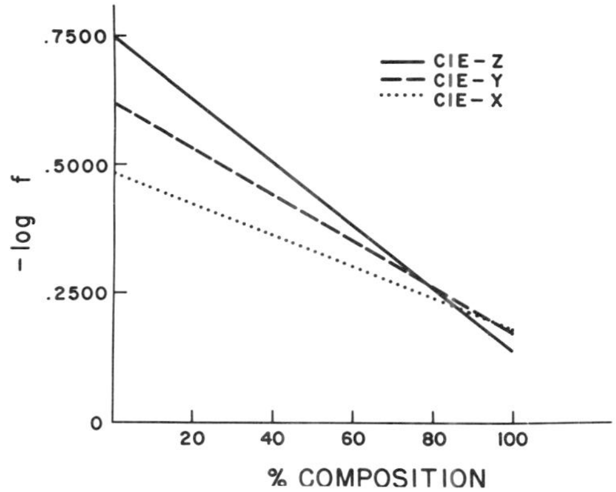

FIG. 3—*A Blending diagram for a rosé and a white wine.*

be made by blending wines however close in color. A master chart can be prepared that provides information for the general case rather than for two specific starting wines. This is possible because for the most part, the –log *R*, –log *G*, and –log *B* values for wines that have not undergone browning will fall on the vertical. For wines that have browned, the –log *B* value will be off the vertical in the direction of increasing absorption and the –log *G* may deviate to lower values indicating loss of anthocyanin pigment. If the points are too far off the perpendicular, the wine is unsuitable for blending purposes as the resultant blend will have an off-color brownish appearance. This is particularly critical with dark red wines where the red pigment hides the browning, which on dilution becomes objectionably apparent.

Because anthocyanin pigments exist as highly colored cations at low pH values, advantage can be taken of the shift in chromaticity coordinates on acidification as a means of estimating anthocyanin content. The magnitude of the shift $(\Delta x^2 + \Delta y^2)^{1/2}$ is directly related to anthocyanin content.

Loss of anthocyanin and increase in browning can also be followed by determining the change in dominant wavelength and excitation purity as measured by thin-layer transreflectometry [*24*].

The analytical process as a predictor of the synthetic process—Thin-layer transreflectometry proved to be more sensitive than the eye in distinguishing color differences among samples known to vary in controlled fashion. Changes in color must be expressed on a three-dimensional basis due to the critical relationship of –log *R* to –log *G* to –log *B*. Because the objective method is far more sensitive to changes induced by browning than is the eye, its usefulness in predicting the appearance of a blend or in following changes with time is indisputable.

These examples should serve to demonstrate that the physical and chemical properties of a food dictate to a significant extent the conditions under which valid measurements can be made for purposes of color evaluation. In turn, information can be extracted from the measurements to give quantitative data pertaining to the physical and chemical state of the system.

Concluding Remarks

The successful application of the principles presented in this report to a variety of problems, all of which can be described as problems in colorimetry of foods, is offered as evidence to refute the several propositions laid down in the proceedings of the 1954 symposium [*12*] and still prevalently accepted. Specifically, arguments have been presented to:

1. Discourage the concept that the CIE specification is an "objective color measurement." It describes a stimulus in terms of a matching combination of light primaries and is thus concerned with metameric or spectrally unlike matches, not reflectance or transmittance characteristics of the object in question. With foods, attention must be given to the latter, not to additive mixtures of stimulus equivalents. Transformations of CIE space to uniform spaces, such as the L, a, b, or U^*, V^*, W^* are even further removed from measurements of physical characteristics of the sample than X, Y, Z or Y, x, y.

2. Question the rationale of using a single number expression of color differences, ΔE, based on differences of colorimetric specifications among samples at a given time or with time for a given sample. With foods, interest should be focussed on why the samples are different and what happens when changes occur. ΔE simply gives an estimate of the magnitude of visually perceived differences, not which dimensions are involved, nor the directions of differences.

3. Refute the idea that instruments "see" the same way that the human eye does. Photoelectric instruments are analytical tools, not "electric eyes" and must be so considered; the visual process is a synthetic one, with color perceived in its totality.

4. Show that the spectrophotometer cannot be considered the ultimate instrument in the evaluation of color of foods. Indeed, the design characteristics of the spectrophotometer may preclude its use in certain cases. The analytical procedure that satisfies the requirements of a particular case defines the "ultimate" instrument in that instance.

In sum, color evaluation as it pertains to foods must be viewed differently from color evaluation of objects manufactured to a color requirement. With foods, let it be stressed once again that interest lies in obtaining measured values that yield information relating to the condition of the food at a given time, not to stimulus characteristics to ensure visual matches whether metameric or not.

References

[*1*] CIE (Commission Internationale de l'Eclairage), *Proceedings 8th Session,* Cambridge 1931, Cambridge University Press, 1932.

[*2*] Hardy, A. C., *Journal of the Optical Society of America,* Vol. 18, No. 1929, p. 96.

[*3*] Hardy, A. C., *Journal of the Optical Society of America,* Vol. 125, No. 1935, p. 305.

[*4*] Hardy, A. C., *Handbook of Colorimetry,* The Technology Press, M.I.T., 1936.

[*5*] Judd, D. W. and Wyszecki, G., *Color in Business, Science and Industry,* Wiley, New York, 1963.

[*6*] Mackinney, G. and Little, A. C., *Color of Foods,* The Avi Publishing Co., Connecticut, 1962.

[*7*] Hunter, R., *Journal of the Optical Society of America,* Vol. 38, 1948, pp. 661, 1094.

[*8*] Wright, W. D., *The Rays are Not Coloured,* Adam Hilger Ltd., London, 1967, Chapter 1.

[*9*] Fox, D. L., *Animal Biochromes and Structural Colours,* Cambridge University Press, 1953.

[*10*] Band, R. V. and Wright, W. D., *Journal of the Optical Society of America,* Vol. 20, 1930, p. 381.

[*11*] Mac Gillivray, J. H., *Proceedings,* The American Society of Horticultural Science, Vol. 35, 1937, p. 630.

[*12*] *Color of Foods–a Symposium,* Advisory Board, Quartermaster Research and Development, National Academy of Science, National Research Council, Washington, D. C., 1954.

[*13*] Mackinney, G., Little, A. C., and Brinner, L., *Food Technology,* Vol. 20, 1966, p. 60.

[*14*] Little, A. C., *Color Engineering,* Vol. 5, 1967, p. 48.

[*15*] Little, A. C., *Die Farbe,* Vol. 14, 1965, p. 148.

[*16*] Little, A. C. and Mackinney, G., *Food Technology,* Vol. 23, 1969, p. 25.

[*17*] Clydesdale, F. M., *Food Technology,* Vol. 26, 1972, p. 45.

[*18*] Little, A. C. and Mackinney, G., *Food Technology,* Vol. 10, 1956, p. 503.

[*19*] Little, A. C., *Journal of Food Science,* Vol. 29, 1964, p. 782.

[*20*] Little, A. C., *Food Technology,* Vol. 23, 1969, p. 71, p. 134, p. 136.

[*21*] Little, A. C., *American Journal of Enology and Viticulture,* Vol. 22, 1971, pp. 138, 144, 203.

[*22*] Association of Official Analytical Chemists, *Official Method of Analysis,* 10th Ed., 1965, p. 131.

[*23*] Little, A. C. and Liaw, M. W., in preparation.

[*24*] Joslyn, M. and Little, A. C., *American Journal of Enology and Viticulture,* Vol. 18, 1967, p. 138.

J. N. Yeatman[1] *and B. B. Aulenbach*[2]

Relationship of Instrumental Measurements to Visual Impressions of Potato Chip Color*

REFERENCE: Yeatman, J. N. and Aulenbach, B. B., "**Relationship of Instrumental Measurements to Visual Impressions of Potato Chip Color,**" *Sensory Evaluation of Appearance of Materials, ASTM STP 545,* American Society for Testing and Materials, 1973, pp. 128-138.

ABSTRACT: A method was developed for preparing flat potato chips suitable for colorimetric measurement and visual evaluation. Flat potato chips were evaluated by three techniques: (1) colorimetric, including and excluding ultraviolet (UV) light in measuring beam to determine fluorescence effects; (2) spectrophotometric (380 to 740 nm), alternately backing chips with black or white reflector to permit calculation of light scattering; (3) visual, under controlled illumination by an experienced panel using a simple color-scoring system.

Excluding UV light increased Hunter a_L and b_L values. Although visual color scores under two luminaires (UV included and UV somewhat attenuated) were similar, greater attenuation of the UV light might affect visual impressions. Visual scores were highly correlated with Hunter L and a_L, indicating that these instrumental measurements could be used to predict visual impressions of chip color. Munsell notations of chip color derived from spectrophotometric measurements backed with white reflector matched Munsell papers better than notations derived from data corrected for light scattering.

Color photographs were made of a series of flat potato chips with a Munsell gray scale in the frame register, permitting precise reproduction of a new visual color guide. The method of flat chip preparation for instrumental measurement and the visual color guide are offered as improved optional procedures in U.S. Standards for Grades of Potatoes for Processing.

KEY WORDS: potatoes, preparation, senses, visual perception, colorimetry, spectrophotometry, Munsell color system, ultraviolet radiation, correlation, fluorescence, perception

*The mention of specific instruments, trade names, or manufacturers is made for the purpose of identification and does not imply any endorsement by the U. S. Government.

[1] Research food technologist, Bureau of Foods, Food and Drug Administration, Washington, D. C. 20204.

[2] Food technologist, Agricultural Research Service, U. S. Department of Agriculture, Beltsville, Md. 20705.

Improved objective methods for grading potatoes for processing and a good visual guide for evaluating chip color have been needed for many years. The color of chips is the main quality attribute influencing consumer acceptability. Smith [*1*],[3] in his extensive review of factors affecting potato quality, points out that high reducing sugar is a primary cause of unacceptably dark chips, which may sometimes be corrected by special treatment before and during processing.

When potatoes are graded according to the revised U. S. Standards for Grades of Potatoes for Processing [*2*], chips are prepared from a sample and compared with a minimum acceptable color, Munsell notation 10YR 7/8. Although this color test is simpler than the method described by O'Keefe [*3*], where samples are compared with photographs of piles of chips, reliance on a single color standard is not satisfactory.

Davis and Smith [*4*] reported that the Agtron® Model F reflectometer provided a rapid, accurate color measurement of potato chips and other processed potato products. However, chips must be crushed before measuring, and the color obtained may not resemble that of intact chips. Findlen and Yeatman [*5*] attempted to develop an improved procedure for preparing chips for evaluation and suggested that factors such as light scatter and fluorescence might affect instrumental measurements.

Our research had the following objectives: (1) to develop a procedure for preparing flat potato chips for direct instrumental color measurement and visual evaluation; (2) to measure color of intact flat chips instrumentally, investigating factors such as fluorescence; and (3) to evaluate flat chip color by a simple visual method and develop a new series of color standards for subjective evaluation.

Procedure

Preliminary Test

The preliminary test was designed to establish the best techniques for chip preparation, instrumental measurement, and visual evaluation to use in more extensive tests. Details on potato varieties and chemical composition will not be given because they were less important than the color of the resulting chips.

Chip Preparation—A critical factor in chip preparation is obtaining slices of uniform thickness. Although use of an inexpensive home-type electric slicer would have been desirable, thickness variation within a slice was much too high, ranging from 0.099 to 0.686 cm. A restaurant-type slicer with constant pressure feed and precise thickness adjustment was used to prepare slices comparable to commercial practice (0.140 ± 0.013 cm). Chips were cut from lengthwise slices with a 5-cm diameter corkborer and fried in 182°C (360°F) cottonseed oil in a home-type thermostatically controlled deep-well cooker.

For direct instrumental measurement, chips must be flat, not curled, as is usual. Each potato disk was fried between two pieces of 0.159-cm mesh

[3] The italic numbers in brackets refer to the list of references appended to this paper.

aluminum screen, fastened together with paper clips (Fig. 1). These "sandwiches" were propped against the sides of the cooker to prevent floating to the surface of the oil. Frying time was varied to produce a wide range of color, and twelve flat chips were chosen for instrumental and visual evaluation.

Instrumental Measurements—Color was measured with a Hunter D25 tristimulus colorimeter (0 to 45 deg geometry, 5-cm diameter aperture and incident beam) equipped with a movable filter to exclude or include ultraviolet (UV) light in the incident beam. A white enamel tile ($L = 95.0$, $a_L = -0.8$, $b_L = 3.2$) was used for standardization. Each chip was backed with a standard gray tile (National Bureau of Standards 65). Spectrophotometric measurements between 380 and 740 nm were made with a Cary Model 14R spectrophotometer equipped with a 25-cm integrating sphere, specular reflectance excluded. To permit calculation of light scatter, chips were backed with a black reflector and then with a white reflector. The reflectors were shallow sample cups covered with either carbon black or the rutile form of titanium dioxide (TiO_2) paint. Details of the Kubelka-Munk analysis for light scattering and the theoretical determination of infinite thickness of sample (thickness at which all light would be reflected) are given by Judd and Wyszecki [*6*]. The application of the Kubelka-Munk analysis to food products has been demonstrated by Gullett et al [*7*].

Visual Evaluation—The twelve flat chips were evaluated by 25 untrained

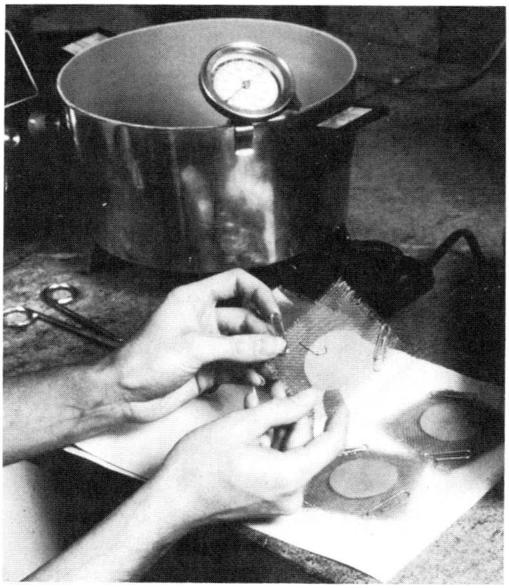

FIG. 1—*Preparation of flat potato chips by frying slices between pieces of aluminum screen.*

panelists under a Macbeth North Sky Daylight (7500 K) Model BBX 324 fixture on three consecutive days. Panelists ranked the chips for lightness and then for "color" (including lightness, hue, and saturation), to see if the results would differ. To establish a color range for the main tests, panelists also ranked the chips by their own color preferences, indicating limits of acceptability.

Main Test

The objectives of the main test were to apply the methods of chip preparation and color evaluation and to develop recommendations for the U. S. Standards for Grades of Potatoes for Processing.

Chip Preparation—A new series of chips was prepared using the same procedures as before, except that oil temperature was 190°C (375°F). Two slices from the same potato were fried simultaneously. One slice was fried as a flat chip and the other was allowed to curl naturally. Varying the frying time from 1 to 10 min produced flat and curly chips in the color range acceptable to the preliminary panel.

Instrumental Measurements—All flat chips were measured with and without UV light in the incident beam on the Hunter D25, using the same procedures as in the preliminary test.

Visual Evaluation—For visual evaluation, two almost identical groups of flat chips (eight chips per group) and their matching curly chips were selected so that each of the four groups formed a gradual color series within the desired range. Selections were based on Hunter L and a_L values of the flat chips, as well as on visual impressions by the junior author. Two additional flat chips, one lighter and the other darker than the series, were chosen as standard endpoints to be viewed with all other chips. Five panelists who performed consistently well in the preliminary test and who scored low (best) on the Farnsworth-Munsell 100 Hue Test made the visual evaluations.

Chips were evaluated under each of two Macbeth Norlite D7500 Model 840 luminaires suspended 66 cm above the viewing surface (intensity of 280 ft candles). One luminaire contained a polished aluminum reflector (UV included). The reflector of the second luminaire was sprayed four times with TiO_2 paint, which somewhat attenuated the UV energy. Light from the luminaires was measured with a Gamma® spectroradiometer equipped with cosine receptor, grating monochromator and S-20 response side-window photomultiplier. Panelists viewed the chips according to ASTM Methods for Visual Evaluation of Color Differences of Opaque Materials (D 1729-68), on coded paper plates painted with Munsell N 8.5 gray on a background of the same color. The viewing angle was 45 deg.

A statistical plan was developed so that each of the 16 flat and 16 curly chips was evaluated three times under each of the two luminaires. Flat and curly chips were always viewed separately. Panelists were presented eight chips at a time, plus the two standard endpoints. First, they ranked the chips for "chip color" between the endpoints, physically arranging them in a color series. Using the endpoint chips as Points 1 and 10 on a 10-point color scale, they scored each chip for color to indicate degree of visual difference between chips. Average color scores for the five panelists over the three replications were calculated for each of the flat and curly chips under each luminaire.

Results

Preliminary Test

Frying potato slices between pieces of aluminum screen prevented curling and produced flat chips suitable for direct instrumental measurement. Light-weight screen did not produce a "waffled" surface on the chips, as did heavier stainless steel plating. Flat chips could be handled gently without special equipment and could be saved, intact, for future reference.

Panelists found the flat chips easy to evaluate visually. The rank order of the twelve chips for lightness and for "color" were very similar, so a general term, "chip color," was used in the main test. Chips most acceptable to the 25 panelists ranged in Hunter L values from about 75 to 60 and in Hunter a_L/b_L ratios from –0.08 to +0.350. These ranges served as guides in preparing chips for the main test.

Kubelka-Munk calculations of colors of chips of infinite thickness showed that there was considerable light scattering in individual flat potato chips. Correction for light scattering resulted in calculated Munsell notations which were a visual mismatch with the samples. Calculated notations based on spectral data of samples backed with white reflector were a visual color match with the samples.

Main Test

Before comparing Hunter values for the 18 flat chips with and without UV in the light beam, values for UV excluded were corrected to remove built-in differences due to instrument standard settings so that remaining differences would be due to effects of excluding UV. Hunter values for one set of eight flat chips and the standard endpoints are shown in Table 1. Values for the second set of flat chips were very similar. Including or excluding UV had no effect upon Hunter L values. When UV was excluded, both a_L and b_L values increased. Chips with higher a_L values should appear yellow-red and redder to the eye. Chips with higher b_L values should appear more saturated in color. Viewed under blacklight (365 nm), the chips fluoresced with an intense blue-white color. When Hunter data were converted to CIE values (Table 1), the Z values indicated that it is the blue end of the spectral reflectance curve which is affected by the presence or absence of UV in the light source, completely compatible with the observed blue-white fluorescence.

TABLE 1—*Colorimeter measurements for one set of flat potato chips (UV included and excluded in incident beam), with CIE conversions.*

Chip	UV included or excluded	Hunter Values[a]			CIE Conversions		
		L	a_L	b_L	*X*	*Y*	*Z*
A[b]	included	78.7	−1.7	19.2	60.0	61.9	47.6
	excluded	78.8	2.5	24.4	62.0	62.1	40.9
B	included	77.0	−0.1	22.8	58.1	59.3	40.4
	excluded	77.2	4.1	27.3	60.2	59.6	34.8
C	included	75.3	1.1	24.7	56.1	56.7	35.6
	excluded	75.8	5.2	28.4	58.5	57.5	31.5
D	included	72.5	2.8	25.3	52.7	52.6	31.1
	excluded	72.8	6.9	28.6	54.8	53.0	27.4
E	included	71.6	2.8	25.1	51.4	51.3	30.2
	excluded	71.5	7.8	29.4	53.2	51.1	24.9
F	included	68.2	5.1	25.8	47.5	46.5	25.2
	excluded	67.8	10.4	30.2	49.0	46.0	19.7
G	included	64.5	7.4	24.2	43.5	41.6	22.8
	excluded	64.8	11.4	27.2	45.3	42.0	19.8
H	included	61.4	8.4	22.8	39.8	37.7	20.9
	excluded	61.5	12.3	26.0	41.3	37.8	17.7
I	included	55.7	10.4	20.5	33.7	31.0	17.4
	excluded	55.9	13.9	23.2	35.0	31.2	15.0
J[b]	included	49.5	11.9	18.4	27.3	24.5	13.6
	excluded	50.3	14.1	20.2	28.8	25.3	12.7

[a] Values corrected to equivalent standardization, UV included.
[b] Standard endpoint chips.

Average color scores for chips viewed under the two luminaires were similar, as shown for flat chips in Fig. 2. Coating the reflector of one luminaire with TiO_2 paint resulted in a slight attenuation of UV energy in the viewing area, not comparable to the large attenuation effected by the UV-excluding filter in the D25 colorimeter (Table 2). More research is needed to evaluate effects of UV light on visual impressions of potato chip color. Similarity of scores under the two luminaires shows that standard endpoints helped panelists to score color consistently under somewhat different conditions of illumination.

Color scores for flat chips and curly chips were highly correlated under both luminaires ($r = +0.97$ for UV included and $+0.93$ for UV excluded). Panelists were able to ignore chip shape and could use the flat standard endpoints as guides for scoring color of curly chips.

Visual scores for flat chips were very highly correlated with Hunter L and a_L values, regardless of UV conditions. Figures 3 and 4 show these relationships for UV included. Visual scores and a_L/b_L ratios were also highly correlated ($r = +0.99$). By using two endpoint chips to anchor the color scale, panelists scored precisely and consistently, contributing to the high correlation coefficients. Based on these results, L or a_L value alone could be used to indicate chip color and predict visual impressions.

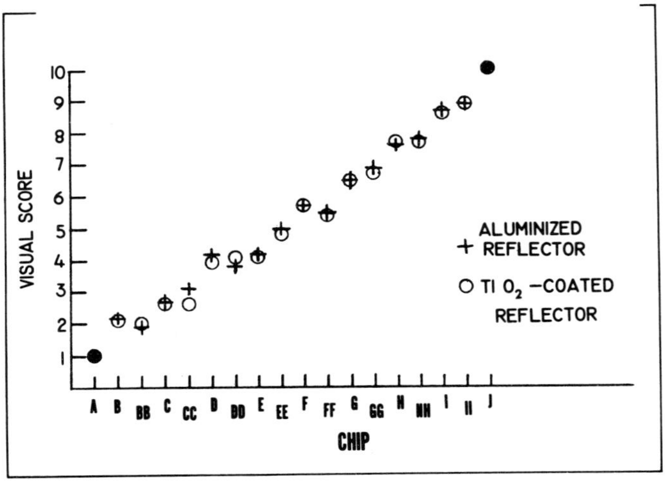

FIG. 2–*Visual color scores for flat potato chips viewed under two luminaires.*

TABLE 2–*Difference in spectral energy distribution of two luminaires (7500 K), with and without ultraviolet attenuation.*[a]

Wavelength, nm[c]	Relative Spectral Energy[b]		Difference in Flux, %
	Lamp 1[d]	Lamp 2[e]	
380	32.5	22.5	−30.8
385	39.3	26.7	−32.1
390	47.3	31.8	−32.8
395	54.6	38.0	−30.4
400	63.0	46.1	−26.8
405	187.7	148.9	−20.7
410	135.1	110.3	−18.4
415	91.0	84.3	−7.4
420	96.1	96.6	+0.5
425	105.2	107.5	+2.1
430	115.9	119.9	+3.3

435-700 nm: Average difference in flux +7.0%

[a] Norlite® 8 tube (1.2 m) fluorescent fixture, 7500 K correlated color temperature.
[b] Gamma® spectroradiometer, with cosine receptor, 560 nm = 100.
[c] Normalized at 560 nm.
[d] Alzak® aluminized reflector, UV included.
[e] Titanium dioxide-coated reflector.

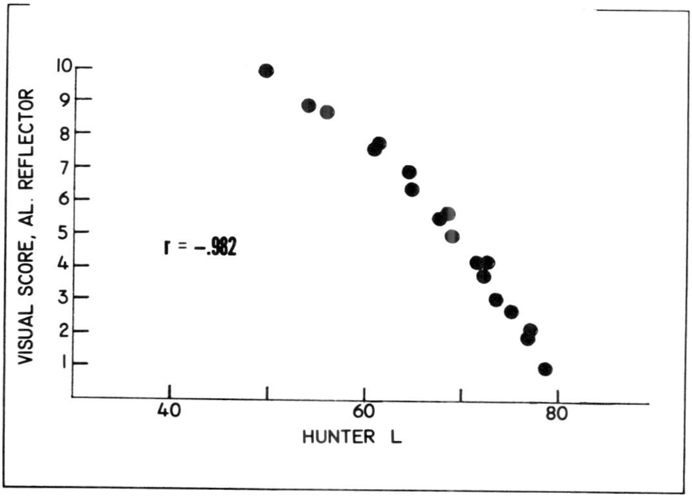

FIG. 3–*Relationship of Hunter L values and visual scores for flat potato chips, UV included.*

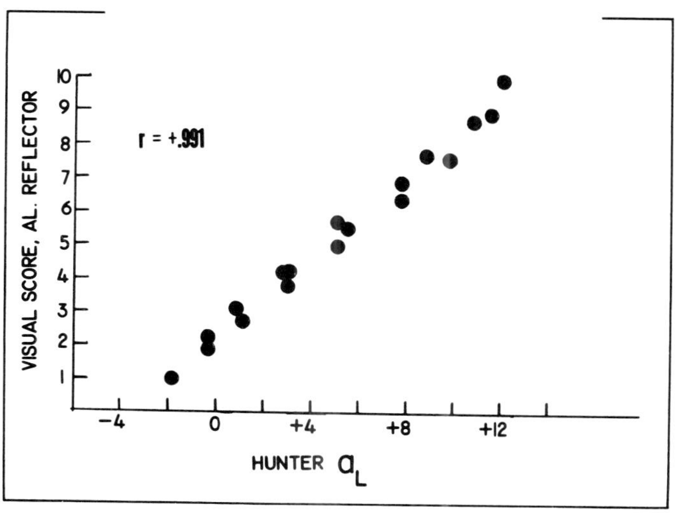

FIG. 4–*Relationship of Hunter a_L values and visual scores for flat potato chips, UV included.*

The relationship between visual scores and b_L values was non-linear (Fig. 5). Because both pale yellow and dark red-brown chips had low b_L values, b_L alone could not be used as an instrumental measurement of chip color. A parabolic regression analysis including the non-linear b_L values, linear a_L values and panelists' scores was calculated. Resulting correlations were, respectively, $R = +0.63$ and $+0.55$ for UV excluded and UV included.

Munsell notations for the colors of the two endpoint chips (A and J) and one series of eight test chips (B through I), shown in Table 3, are based on Hunter L, a_L, and b_L values, UV included, converted to X_{CIE}, Y_{CIE}, and Z_{CIE} values. The color designations in Table 3 also represent the colors of chips in Fig. 6. The color of the chips progressed gradually from a light yellow to a yellow-red.

Munsell notations for a chip that visually matched Chip F (Table 3) were calculated from spectral reflectance curves derived from Kubelka-Munk analysis. Trichromatic coefficients X_{CIE}, Y_{CIE}, and Z_{CIE} were also calculated from spectral data for the same chip backed with white (TiO_2) reflector. The Munsell notation for the chip backed with white (0.9Y 7.1/5.1) was a closer match to Chip F than was the notation (10YR 6.4/4.5) derived from data corrected for light scattering. This finding agrees with results in the preliminary test.

We recommend that the potato chip preparation procedure and the colorimetric measurement of flat chips be included for optional use in the U.S. Standards for Grades of Potatoes for Processing.

The series of flat chips shown in Fig. 6 were photographed in color with a

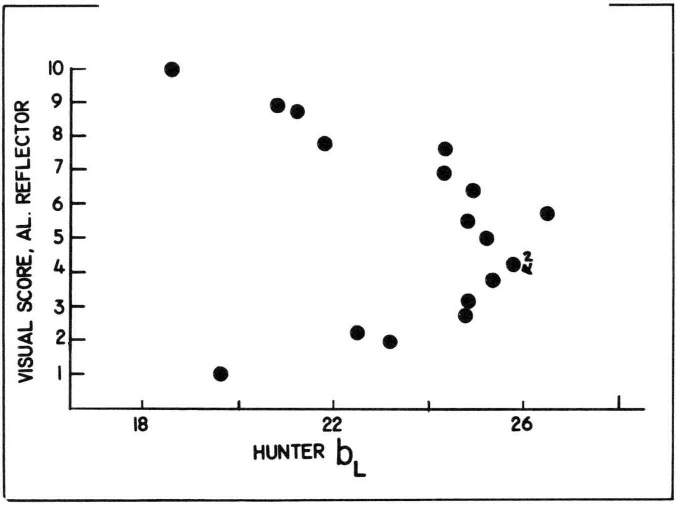

FIG. 5–*Relationship of Hunter b_L values and visual scores for flat potato chips, UV included.*

TABLE 3–*Munsell notations for colors of one set of flat chips in main test.*[a]

Chip	Munsell Notation (Hue, Value/Chroma)
A[b]	3.9Y 8.2/3.1
B	2.9Y 8.0/3.9
C	2.3Y 7.9/4.6
D	1.6Y 7.6/5.1
E	1.4Y 7.5/5.1
F	0.6Y 7.3/5.6
G	9.1YR 6.9/5.7
H	8.3YR 6.6/6.0
I	7.2YR 6.1/5.6
J[b]	5.7YR 5.5/5.4

[a] Calculated from Hunter L, a_L, and b_L (UV included) converted to X, Y, and Z.
[b] Standard endpoint chips.

Munsell gray scale in the frame register, permitting precise color photographic reproduction. The colors of these chips are more realistic than those in another widely used photograph [*3*]. The Munsell notations of the chips (Table 3) define their colors in psychophysical terms. Because visual color scores and instrumental color of these chips were so highly correlated, we recommend this photograph in color as a new visual guide for chip color evaluation.

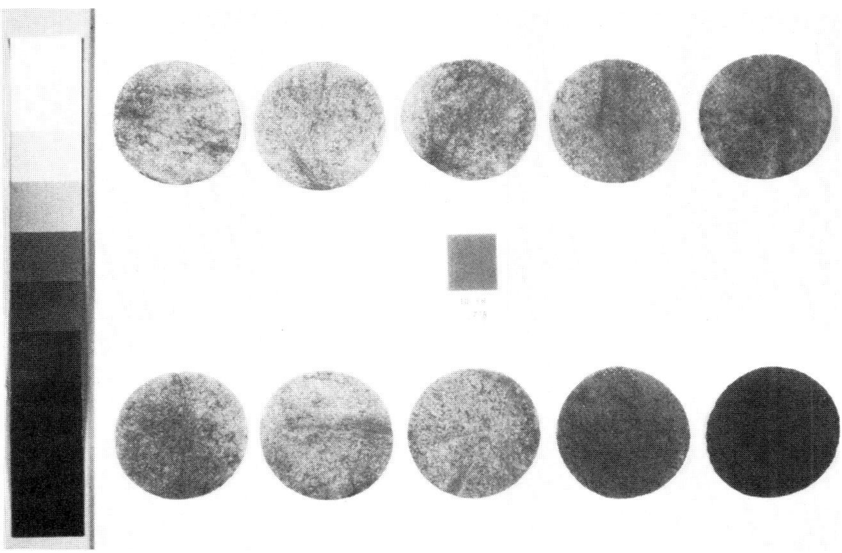

FIG. 6–*Series of ten flat potato chips offered as new visual guide for chip color evaluation.*

References

[*1*] Smith, Ora in *1966 Frontiers of Food Research Symposium Proceedings,* Cornell University Press, Ithaca, N. Y., 1966, pp. 5-29.

[*2*] "United States Standards for Grades of Potatoes for Processing," Agricultural Marketing Service, U. S. Department of Agriculture, 1963, Title 7, Sections 51.3410-51.3424.

[*3*] O'Keefe, R. G., *Nebraska Experiment Station Quarterly,* Lincoln, Vol. 17, No. 3, Fall 1970, pp. 16-17.

[*4*] Davis, C. O. and Smith, Ora, *Potato Chipper,* Vol. 21, No. 11, Nov. 1962, pp. 72-76.

[*5*] Findlen, Herbert and Yeatman, J. N., *Proceedings,* 17th National Potato Utilization Conference, 1967, pp. 52-56.

[*6*] Judd, D. B. and Wyszecki, Gunter, *Color in Business, Science, and Industry,* 2nd ed., Wiley, New York, 1963, pp. 387-405.

[*7*] Gullett, E. A., Francis, F. J., and Clydesdale, F. M., *Journal of Food Science,* Vol. 37, No. 3, 1972, pp. 389-393.

P. E. Green [1]

Measurement of Judgmental Responses to Multi-Attribute Marketing Stimuli

REFERENCE: Green, P. E., "**Measurement of Judgmental Responses to Multi-Attribute Marketing Stimuli,**" *Sensory Evaluation of Appearance of Materials, ASTM STP 545,* American Society for Testing and Materials, 1973, pp. 139-153.

ABSTRACT: A set of three interrelated research designs are presented and solutions are illustrated with synthetic data. The problems include (*a*) measuring the relative importance of a group of product benefits, (*b*) selecting a package design that best connotes the psychological imagery of a subset of the selected benefits, and (*c*) determining what point-of-purchase display materials, brand name, and brand pricing strategy to employ in initial market introduction. Structurally, all three problems involve non-numerical, judgmental responses to multi-attribute marketing stimuli.

All three problems are "solved" by conjoint measurement. This approach, recently developed in mathematical psychology, draws upon previous work in experimental design, unidimensional psychophysics and data theory. The paper concludes with a discussion of current limitations of the approach and potential marketing application areas.

KEY WORDS: senses, perception, stimulus (psychophysiology), marketing, design

The pretesting of product benefit combinations, package designs, brand-price combinations, advertisements, special offers—indeed, almost any type of marketing stimulus—is typically beset by the following complexities.

1. The response variable is often expressed in a judgmental, perhaps even mood-like form. For example, which dessert package best connotes the characteristics of "light and tangy," which product-price combination suggests the best "value for money," which advertisement has the greatest "attention-getting value"?

2. The stimuli are multi-attribute in nature, for example, packages may vary

[1] S. S. Kresge Professor of Marketing, Wharton School, University of Pennsylvania, Philadelphia, Pa. 19104.

in size, color, shape, logotype; print advertisements may differ in amount of white space, proportion of area devoted to pictorial material, type of copy appeal, and so on.

3. The researcher is often ignorant of not only the partial contribution that each attribute level of the stimulus makes to the total psychological response but also the appropriate "objective" scales by which the attributes themselves are to be measured.

4. The partial contributions of attribute levels may interact—the psychological effect of lighter shades of yellow on the response, "light and tangy," may depend on the shape of the dessert package.

The pervasive nature of judgmental evaluation problems that involve multi-attribute stimuli under poorly understood response conditions and the desire to develop "lexicons," that is, types of dictionaries that, in principle, could translate changes in physical variables to psychological responses of interest (for example, preference) has motivated the research design underlying this report.

In brief, the author will take the view that complex, judgmental responses to multi-attribute stimuli can sometimes be decomposed into partial contributions that are psychophysical, namely, related to physical or other objective changes in a set of controllable variables. This decomposition-like approach shares the same kinds of limitations that all reductionist approaches exhibit. Still it may be useful from both pragmatic (Which package design should be implemented now?) and theoretical (How does one go about designing packages in the first place?) points of view.

The antecedents of the research discussed here are primarily drawn from three areas: (*a*) the experimental design literature, particularly those aspects involving response-surface methods [*1,2*];[2] (*b*) the contributions of the classical psychophysicists [*3*]; and (*c*) the literature of data theory, especially those facets that deal with ranking or categorical responses to multi-attribute stimuli [*4*].

Collectively, these antecedents have provided the background for the development of a new methodology that is known as "conjoint measurement." Conjoint measurement is concerned with determining the separate (and, in this case, psychological) contributions of a set of independent variables to the ordering (or possibly, mere categorization) of a dependent variable. These partial contributions and the dependent variable can be conjointly measured (asymptotically) at the level of separate interval scales with common unit even though the response variable is (originally) non-numerical. As such, one can obtain psychological scale transformations of the objective independent variables—multidimensional psychophysical scales, as it were—from nonnumerical psychological responses to the multi-attribute stimuli.

[2] The italic numbers in brackets refer to the list of references appended to this paper.

Research Problems

In order to motivate the discussion, our research design is couched in terms of an actual marketing situation concerning three (illustrative) problems.

1. What combination of product benefits[5] should be implemented in the form of a new product by a producer of self-polishing floor waxes?

2. Having settled on a product formulation that effects certain consumer benefits, what type of package should be designed to connote these benefits?

3. What brand name-price-display-appeals combination should be selected for market introduction?

Since some aspects of the methodology may be unfamiliar to the reader, each of the above problems is illustrated in terms of synthetic (and highly simplified) data. Following a discussion of each of these interrelated problems, we describe some of the limitations of the approach and conclude the report by suggesting some possible areas of application in marketing research.

In the course of describing each of the three research problems, some of the conceptual aspects of conjoint measurement will be discussed, although no detailed mathematical statement is attempted here. Interested readers should see Refs *6-8*.

Product Benefits Evaluation

We first assume that the analyst has assembled, by more or less conventional marketing research approaches, a list of self-polishing floor wax user benefits that are thought to be considered the most important to the market, as considered generically. These benefits appear in the upper panel of Table 1. Unknown to the researcher, the "average" consumer values the presence of each of these benefits according to the numerical scale values ("utilities") shown in the upper panel of Table 1.

The researcher is interested in finding out what these scale values are, not considered only separately (since interactions could exist) but, rather in various combinations. Each of the benefits can be characterized as a qualitative factor in a 2^5 factorial design where each benefit is either present or absent (assumed in the latter case to result in a zero contribution to consumer utility).

Suppose the researcher feels that one or more two-factor (but no higher order) interactions might exist. The fractional factorial design[9] shown in the lower panel of Table 1 permits one to estimate, with only 16 rather than 32 observations, all main effects and two-factor interactions. Since the researcher assumes that all of the benefits contribute some positive utility, he can also omit the null combination, coded (1), leading to only 15 combinations of benefits. In this case the 15 combinations are made up of all distinct pairs (10 in number) and all distinct quadruples (5 in number).

At this point it is apparent that we have developed a more or less traditional

TABLE 1–*Self-polishing floor wax benefits, scale values and accompanying fractional factorial design (Problem 1).*

	Product Benefit	Utility Scale Value
A.	Resists scuffing, soiling and wear	3.6
B.	Brings floor up to a high, clear gloss	1.0
C.	Resists water and detergent spotting	2.7
D.	Resists skidding and yellowing	0.7
E.	Pleasant scented and easy to apply	1.5

Fractional Factorial Design–Factor Level: Present (1) or Absent (0)

Combination	A	B	C	D	E	Rank
(1)	0	0	0	0	0	(not included)
ae	1	0	0	0	1	9
be	0	1	0	0	1	3
ab	1	1	0	0	0	8
ce	0	0	1	0	1	6
ac	1	0	1	0	0	11
bc	0	1	1	0	0	5
abce	1	1	1	0	1	15[a]
de	0	0	0	1	1	2
ad	1	0	0	1	0	7
bd	0	1	0	1	0	1
abde	1	1	0	1	1	12
cd	0	0	1	1	0	4
acde	1	0	1	1	1	14
bcde	0	1	1	1	1	10
abcd	1	1	1	1	0	13

[a] Denotes top-ranked combination.

fractional factorial design. However, the researcher feels that the respondent, at best, can only "rank order" the 15 benefit combinations from "like best" (Rank 15) to "like least" (Rank 1). Here is where one departs from traditional analysis of variance procedures, which typically assume a numerically valued response variable.

Conjoint measurement algorithms, on the other hand, require only rank order (in some cases only unordered categorical) responses, yet yield (asymptotically) interval scaled values for the partial contributions of each factor level. They accomplish this task by finding, iteratively, a monotone function of the response variable whose (interval scaled) values are most concordant with the prespecified model.[3]

Applying Conjoint Measurement

Suppose, unknown to the researcher, that a respondent does have the utility scale values shown in Table 1. That is, while she cannot explicate them she

[3] That is, minimize a (normalized) residual sums of squares between the fitted parameter values of the model and the numerical values of the (best-fitting) monotone transformation of the original data.

behaves toward the 15 combinations of benefits as though each benefit is separately scaled, as shown in the upper panel of Table 1. Moreover, we assume that her model is a simple additive utility model. That is, the psychological value of any benefit combination is merely the sum of the component utilities making up the combination.

If she behaves this way, then she would give the ranking for the various benefit combinations that appears in the lower panel of Table 1. Although the researcher has developed a fractional factorial design (capable of estimating all main effects and two-factor interactions), let us also assume that he decides to try an additive utility model first. One of the conjoint measurement algorithms, MONANOVA[*10*], is expressly designed for factorial designs utilizing additive models. This algorithm finds both the scale values of each factor level and the best fitting monotone transformation whose values can be expressed as additive combinations of the separate factor contributions.

This algorithm was applied to the synthetic data (the ranks) shown in the lower panel of Table 1. In this error-free case the program required only two iterations to achieve a solution. The upper panel of Fig. 1 shows a plot of the scale values found by MONANOVA against the original (synthetic data) scale values, while the lower panel shows the best fitting monotone transform of the fitted (additive) model versus the original rank order data.

Clearly, in this errorless case the algorithm does quite well, as evinced by the almost linear plot between derived scale values and the original scale values. Given this kind of result, the researcher would not need to try more elaborate, interaction-type models (although we discuss this case subsequently). Thus he has (*a*) established the fact that a main-effects, additive model applies and (*b*) found the psychological component utilities (with common unit) associated with each product benefit. Given the applicability of the additive model, he could deduce the subjective (consumer) ordering of any comparisons involving combinations of the five product benefits. In brief, he has measured the contributions of the independent variables *and* the dependent variable.

Note further that the model can be applied to the responses of a single individual. Realistically speaking, if more than a single respondent is involved, separate scales can be obtained for each or, if desired, the data for all respondents may be scaled as replications. We would favor the former approach as a way to examine individual differences in utility functions—differences that might be related to other respondent characteristics, for example, demographic, socioeconomic, or life style. Conjoint measurement, coupled with clustering techniques[*11*] could provide a way to segment respondents on the basis of commonality of utilities for the various benefit combinations.

In brief, then, we have demonstrated how conjoint measurement can be applied to a 2^5 factorial design (actually a fractional factorial) in which all factors are qualitative and where no error has been explicitly introduced. In this

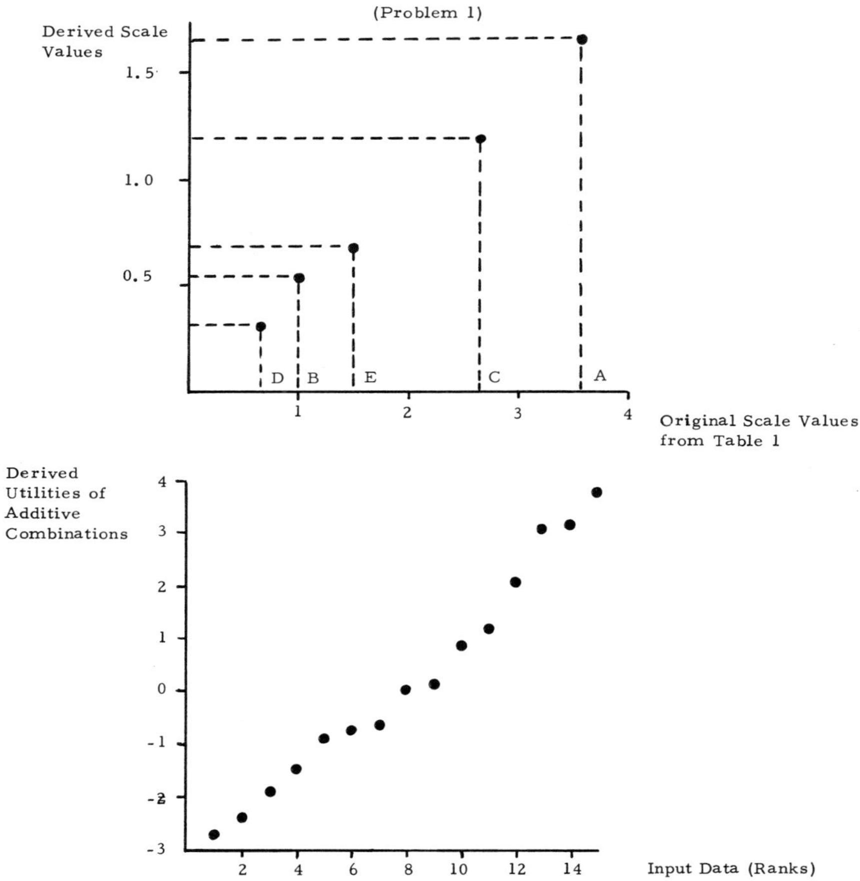

FIG. 1–*Plot of derived versus original scales–fractional fractorial design.*

simplified case the model was a main-effects, additive one. The derived scales could be used to predict share of choices for preference comparisons involving any mixed combination–singles, pairs, triples, quadruples–of the product benefits by summing the separately obtained utility values of each respondent or, more pragmatically, of averaged scale values of respondent clusters that exhibit similar response characteristics.

Package Design Evaluation

We now turn to Problem 2, a situation that differs both substantively and structurally from the preceding one. We assume that the researcher has settled upon two product benefits that are both appealing to a specific market segment and technically feasible to implement.[4] These benefits are assumed to be (*a*) resists scuffing, soiling and wear and (*b*) resists water and detergent spotting. The problem now is to design a package for the product that best connotes these claims from a psychological standpoint. We further assume, for the sake of simplicity, that only three physical variables—(1) shade of blue background color, light to dark, (2) ratio of height to diameter of cylindrical metal container, and (3) diameter of pouring spout—are the control variables of interest. Other variables are controlled at standard levels.

From a structural standpoint, the factors are all quantitative. We assume that four levels of each factor are being considered, leading to a 4^3 design of 64 possible combinations. Here, however, the researcher is reasonably sure that a main-effects model applies; hence, he desires to employ another type of fractional factorial—in this case a Latin square design (lower panel of Fig. 2)—for estimating main effects on the basis of only 16 combinations [*12*].

Unknown to the researcher, the average respondent of the target segment exhibits the psychophysical transforms shown in the upper panel of Fig. 2 for each of the physical variables. Again, she cannot explicate these functions but is assumed to behave as though the functions summarize her psychological reaction to the various combinations. However, any specific respondent is assumed to obey the average configuration with the addition of an error term (assumed to be normally and independently distributed with mean zero and a standard deviation of 0.25) applied at the individual cell level. We assume that 15 respondents, in total, participate in this experiment.

In setting up the experiment the researcher enlists the aid of a commercial artist who prepares 16 package designs, according to the Latin square display shown in the lower panel of Fig. 2. These 16 designs are photographed in color and presented to each respondent. The respondent is asked to rank the designs from the one that most connotes the benefits, "resists scuffing, soiling, wear, water and detergent spotting," to the one that least seems to connote these appeals.

What the researcher receives is a rank order from each of the 15 respondents. Given the presence of error, these rank orders differ across subjects. Again, for purposes of simplification, we assume that the researcher wants to apply conjoint measurement only to the rankings aggregated over the 15 respondents. These group ranks appear in the lower panel of Fig. 2.

In the present case the input data, representing the aggregate rankings, arranged as a fractional factorial, were read in as part of a full factorial design

[4] In this regard one could have also conducted a prior test in which the respondent is asked to order the various benefit combinations utilized in the previous example in terms of believability, that is, her judgment that a single product could "make good" on each combination of benefit claims.

(Problem 2)

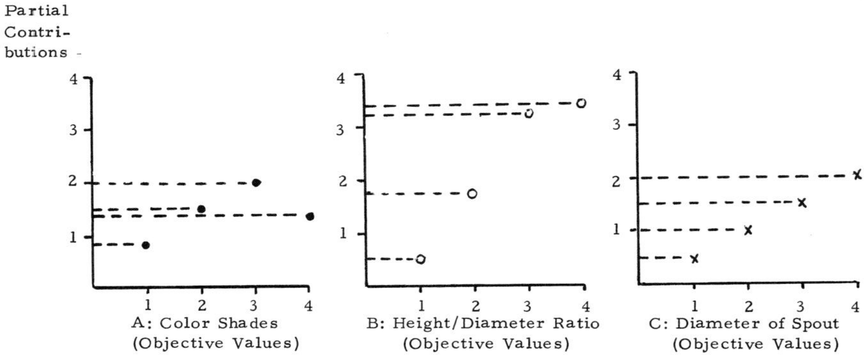

Latin Square Design

Factor A	Factor B 1	2	3	4
1	C_1(1)*	C_2 (3)	C_4 (11)	C_3 (10)
2	C_2 (2)	C_3 (7)	C_1 (8)	C_4 (16)
3	C_3(6)	C_4 (12)	C_2 (15)	C_1 (9)
4	C_4(5)	C_1 (4)	C_3 (14)	C_2 (13)

( )* Response Ranks -- "16" denotes top-ranked combination

FIG. 2–*Partial contributions of package design variables to imagery of selected product benefits and accompanying Latin square design.*

and the missing data feature of the MONANOVA program was used. Figure 3 shows the partial contribution scales obtained from this algorithm. The derived scales are plotted against the actual scales (obtained from projections onto the vertical axes of Fig. 2). While the scatter plots do not show perfect linear plots–in view of the added error term–the recovery is still rather remarkable, given data for only 16 out of a possible 64 observations. The function associated with Factor C (diameter of spout) is the only one that departs much at all from linearity. Thus, even in the presence of moderate amounts of error, the partial contributions are still recovered reasonably well.

Brand Name-Price-Display Evaluation

In the third illustrative problem, we assume that the researcher has settled on the "best" combination of package design variables but now wishes to test the

(Problem 2)

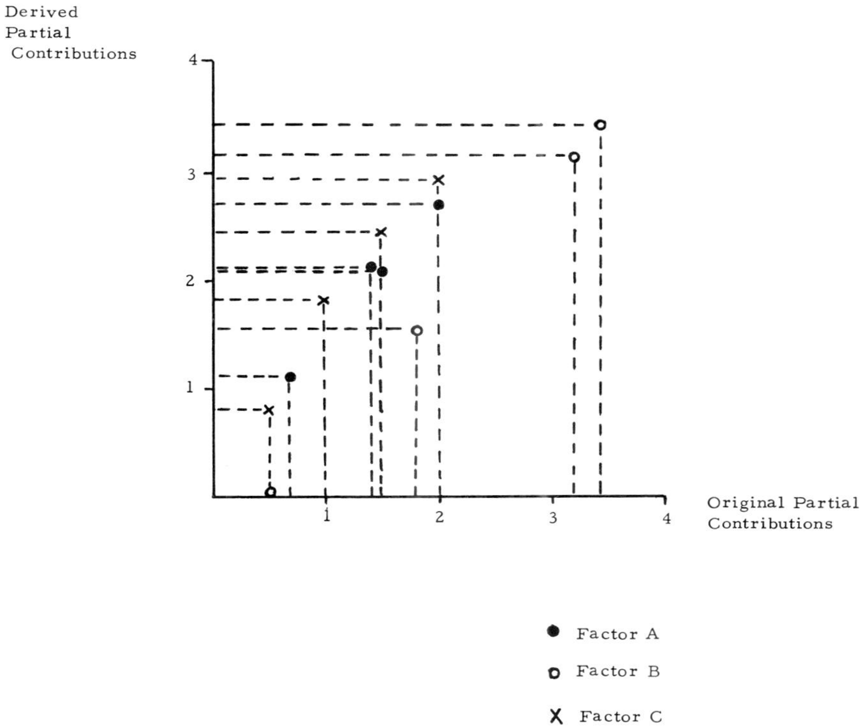

FIG. 3–*Plot of derived versus original partial contributions–Latin square design.*

effect of brand name, price, and display material on overall consumer evaluation, namely, preference.[5] Again, for purposes of simplification, we assume that four factors, each at two levels, are under consideration: (*a*) two brand names; (*b*) two levels of price–one at current average market and one that is 10 percent lower; (*c*) two sizes of display rack; and (*d*) two types of point-of-purchase appeals.

Structurally, we deal here with a mixed (qualitative-quantitative) 2^4 full

[5] We assume, perhaps unrealistically, that the "best" combination of package design variables remains best in the context of brand name, price, display, and copy material. Otherwise, a larger experiment encompassing all of these variables would, of course, be required. By using efficient, for example, fractional factorial designs, such large experiments are feasible without placing an undue judgmental burden on the respondent.

factorial design, consisting of 16 combinations. While, for expository purposes, no error is introduced, we now assume that Factors B (price) and C (size of display rack) interact, that is, if price is below market and the display rack is large, the effect on evaluation involves multiplication of their separate partial contributions in addition to their single factor-level effects. The single factor-level effects and the implied rank order of responses (reflecting the interaction term) appear in Fig. 4.

PREFMAP[*13*], a type of conjoint measurement algorithm that is suitable for dealing with interaction terms, was employed in this problem. This algorithm utilizes dummy-variable coding and, hence, treats analysis of variance computations within a generalized regression framework. In this case, however, the

(Problem 3)

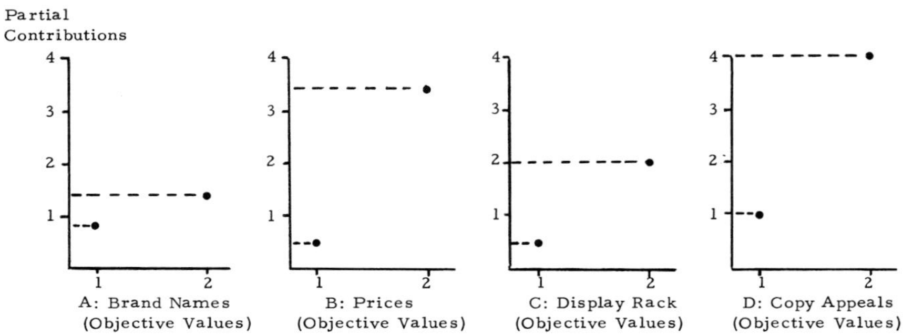

Full Factorial Design: Levels 1 (0) and 2 (1)

Combination	A	B	C	D	BC	Rank
(1)	0	0	0	0	0	1
d	0	0	0	1	0	6
c	0	0	1	0	0	3
cd	0	0	1	1	0	9
b	0	1	0	0	0	5
bd	0	1	0	1	0	11
bc	0	1	1	0	1	13
bcd	0	1	1	1	1	15
a	1	0	0	0	0	2
ad	1	0	0	1	0	8
ac	1	0	1	0	0	4
acd	1	0	1	1	0	10
ab	1	1	0	0	0	7
abd	1	1	0	1	0	12
abc	1	1	1	0	1	14
abcd	1	1	1	1	1	16*

16* Denotes top-ranked combination

FIG. 4–*Partial contributions of brand name, price, display rack, and copy appeals to overall evaluation and accompanying full factorial design.*

regression is monotone rather than linear. The multiplicative interaction term for Factors B and C is merely introduced as an additional zero-one predictor, as shown in the lower panel of Fig. 4.

Figure 5 shows the results of this analysis. The horizontal axis represents the increment between the first and second levels of each original partial-contribution scale (see vertical axis projections in Fig. 4). The vertical axis of Fig. 5 represents the scale values (derived from PREFMAP) for the second level of each factor. As noted, the interaction term is 3.4 × 2 = 6.8 when Factors B and C are each at their second level and zero when these factors are at their first level. Again we observe the high linearity between original and derived scales, indicating that conjoint measurement can cope with interaction terms as well as with main effects.

Finally, we briefly consider the case in which it is assumed that the respondent can only categorize responses—"like very much" to "like very little."

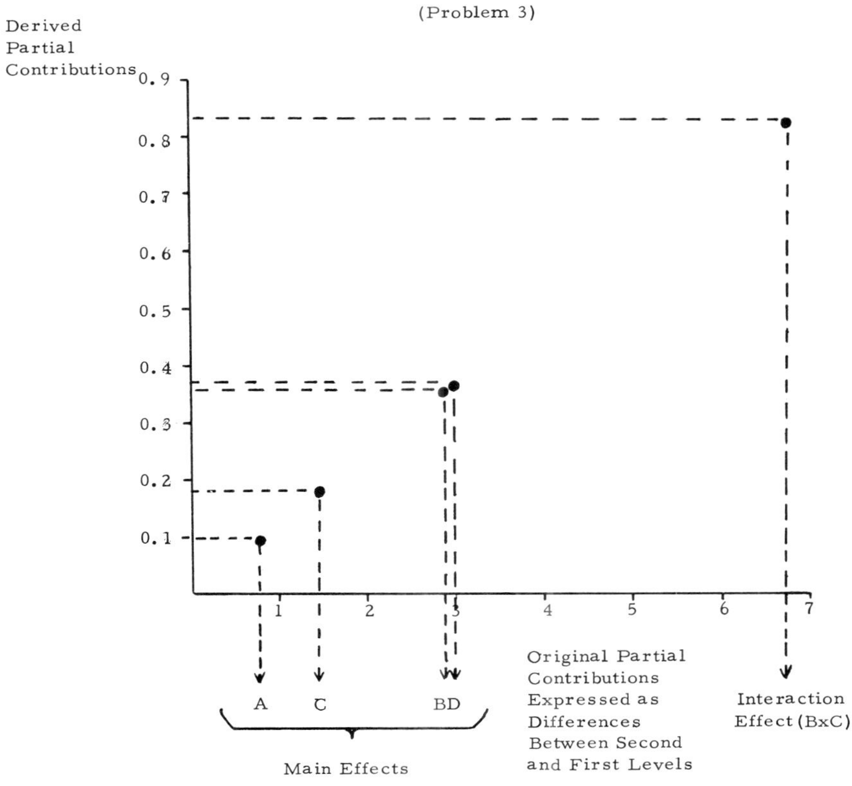

FIG. 5–*Plot of derived versus original partial contributions–full factorial design.*

While we might feel that such descriptive categories can be ordered *a priori* by appropriate choice of adjectival phases, occasions can arise in which the researcher might want to test this assumption. Categorical Conjoint Measurement [*14*] is appropriate for either the ordered category or unordered category case. However, like MONANOVA, this algorithm fits only main-effects, additive models.

Data for Categorical Conjoint Measurement were simulated by partitioning the 16 ranks of Fig. 4 (lower panel) into four categories. Due to space limitations, we do not show the results of this algorithm. But it is of interest to report that Categorical Conjoint Measurement, even in the presence of the interaction effect, proceeded to find numerical values for the four categories that preserved their (*a priori* known) rank order.[6]

Categorical Conjoint Measurement oridnarily would be used when the response variable is not known *a priori* to be rank ordered (as is assumed by MONANOVA and PREFMAP). As such, it can be useful in cases where respondents might be asked, for example, to sort various types of package designs into unordered groups, for example, suitable for everyday use, special occasion, gift giving, and so on.

Additional Considerations

In brief, we have described a variety of experiments—qualitative, quantitative, and mixed factors, responses with and without error, additive, interactive models—that are all characterized as embeddable in factorial designs. Partial contributions of the factors to the response variable need not be monotone (for example, Problem 2), let alone linear. In addition, all response variables can be non-numerical, that is, rank orders or categorical responses. Three different conjoint measurement algorithms have been briefly described to illustrate the approach.

In principle, one could utilize the approaches described earlier for any type of factorial data at the level, if desired, of individual subject responses. If more complex designs are utilized, rating scales could be used rather than ranking responses. Only the ordinal properties of such scales are needed for the MONANOVA and PREFMAP[7] algorithms, while only (unordered) categorical responses are needed for Categorical Conjoint Measurement.

Thus, conjoint measurement provides a way to generalize factorial-type designs to non-numerical responses. More importantly, the procedures, taken collectively, provide a generalization of psychophysical procedures to cases

[6] However, partially due to the interaction term, Categorical Conjoint Measurement did not "recover" the original partial contributions (vertical axis projections of Fig. 4) very well. This, of course, emphasizes the need for appropriate model selection.

[7] While not discussed here, the PREFMAP algorithm is also capable of dealing with one or more covariates.

involving multi-attribute stimuli. Through specification of a combinatorial (that is, factorial) model, one can develop interval-scale values for independent and dependent variables conjointly from non-numerical response data. This is one reason why Luce and Tukey [*7*] have termed conjoint measurement a "new type of fundamental measurement," a type that has particular value to psychology and, not inconsequentially, to marketing research as well.

Current Limitations

This is not to say, however, that the approach is without limitations. First, no statistical inferential apparatus, comparable to analysis of variance procedures, currently exists. This drawback hampers appropriate model specification, particularly where interaction terms are involved. As it stands now, changes in goodness of fit as related to additional parameters, can be considered only from a descriptive standpoint, for example, rank correlation between original data and values predicted by the model.

Second, neither conjoint measurement, nor conventional experimental design procedures for that matter, provide help on the selection of appropriate experimental factors in the first place. In areas like new product and package design, the possible factors may greatly exceed time and financial constraints. In such cases one may resort to sequential designs not unlike those employed in response surface methods [*1,2*]. In this case the respondent serves as a psychological "transducer" whose responses are analogous to such physical variables as "yield" of a chemical process.

In addition, however, no appropriate physical scales may exist, that is, researchers may not be able to relate various esthetic qualities—flavor, fluffiness of texture—to "objective" controllable variables. That is, factor levels themselves may be represented by subjective scales, either those of experts or those of the consumer herself. However, one can still find appropriate "psycho-psychological" transforms that may be of interest in predicting some "overall" response to subjective scale values, as considered in combination.

Finally, we are assuming that consumers find it more natural to order or to categorize responses than to provide direct numerical response information and that ordinal or categorical responses would exhibit higher interoccasion reliability than numerical responses. While conjoint measurement is available to deal with non-numerical responses, the question is still moot regarding subjects' abilities to provide reliable numerical data in the first place.

Current Practice

Current applications of conjoint measurement to marketing research is only in the beginning stages. Pilot level applications have been made by the author and his colleagues in the food and housewares field with "reasonable" results. These applications have involved problems in product design, product appeals evaluation, package design, and price-demand relationships. It is still much too early, however, to gauge the effectiveness of these methods versus more conventional procedures. What does seem apparent is the large variety of marketing research problems that could be amenable to these techniques.

Potential Marketing Applications

A number of possible marketing applications of conjoint measurement have already been described in the literature [*15*]. To that list might be added a few other illustrative applications—to be sure, quite tentative and speculative at this time.

Testimonial Advertising

The practice of testimonial advertising usually assumes some congruence between celebrity and product—Arthur Godfrey for Axion, Dick Van Dyke for Kodak. Conjoint measurement could be used to measure the contributions that various celebrity-product-copy combinations make to commercial effectiveness, believability, recall, and so on. In principle, this approach could be extended to cope with product-program-message congruence.

Labeling Information

Another area of possible application concerns the type of information (and how it is to be displayed) to be included on brand labels. Since information retention may be affected by product class-display interaction and differences in consumer interest and knowledge, a rather elaborate design that includes covariates may be required. Still the possibilities for providing guidance for consumerism-type studies appear suggestive enough to consider at least small-scale studies in this area.

Managerial Utility Functions

Although emphasis here has been placed on consumer evaluation functions, some of the same techniques could be used to ascertain managers' part-worth utility functions for various multi-attribute alternatives, for example, store site locations (characterized by differences in land costs, market accessibility, tax structures, etc.); investment alternatives (characterized by differences in risk, average return, compatibility with present activities); evaluations of sales applicants (characterized by differences in work experience, age, education level), and so on. These problems are all similar structurally and require "trade-offs" to be made among conflicting objectives. It is these implicit trade-offs that can be measured by the approaches described here.

Public Service Activities

With increasing corporate interest in social issues—all of which can be characterized as multi-attribute insofar as their effects on various sectors of the economy are concerned—conjoint measurement might also be utilized to examine differences in utility functions for various participants such as government agencies, corporate officers, employees, and consumers. This approach has already been applied on a more narrow and small-scale basis in the examination of differences among the perceptions of management, salesmen, customers, and equipment specifiers for a firm engaged in computer manufacture.

Conclusion

It is not difficult to imagine other possible applications dealing with multi-attribute choice or, for that matter, choices among various collections of items. Conjoint measurement and related techniques dealing with the scaling of similarities and preference data may provide ways to quantify many kinds of judgments that have been viewed historically as qualitative and intangible. Much remains to be done at the empirical, technical, and conceptual levels before the (usually inappropriate and always pretentious) label of "powerful new technique" will be ineluctably applied. But by that time, the more thoughtful researcher will have made his own tests and evaluations.

References

[*1*] Myers, R. S., *Response Surface Methodology,* Allyn & Bacon, Boston, 1971.
[*2*] Wilde, D. J., *Optimum Seeking Methods,* Prentice-Hall, Inc., Englewood Cliffs, N. J., 1964.
[*3*] Guilford, J. P., *Psychometric Methods,* McGraw-Hill Book Co., New York, 1954.
[*4*] Coombs, C. H., *A Theory of Data,* Wiley, New York, 1964.
[*5*] Haley, R. I., *Journal of Marketing,* Vol. 32, July 1968, pp. 30-35.
[*6*] Coombs, C. H., Dawes, R. M., and Tversky, Amos, *Mathematical Psychology: An Elementary Introduction,* Prentice-Hall, Inc., Englewood Cliffs, N. J., 1970.
[*7*] Luce, R. D. and Tukey, J. W., *Journal of Mathematical Psychology,* Vol. 1, 1964, pp. 1-27.
[*8*] Tversky, Amos, *Journal of Mathematical Psychology,* Vol. 4, 1967, pp. 1-20.
[*9*] Winer, B. J., *Statistical Principles in Experimental Design,* McGraw-Hill Book Co., New York, 1962.
[*10*] Kruskal, J. B., *Journal of the Royal Statistical Society,* Series B, Vol. 27, 1965, pp. 251-263.
[*11*] Green, P. E. and Tull, D. S., *Research for Marketing Decisions,* 2nd ed, Prentice-Hall, Inc., Englewood Cliffs, N. J., 1970.
[*12*] Banks, Seymour, *Experimentation in Marketing,* McGraw-Hill Book Co., New York, 1965.
[*13*] Carroll, J. D., "Individual Differences and Multidimensional Scaling," Bell Telephone Laboratories, Murray Hill, N. J., 1969.
[*14*] Carroll, J. D., "Categorical Conjoint Measurement," Bell Telephone Laboratories, Murray Hill, N. J., 1969.
[*15*] Green, P. E. and Rao, V. R., *Journal of Marketing Research,* Vol. 8, Aug. 1971, pp. 355-363.

E. P. Rubacky [1]

Appearance: Likes and Dislikes

REFERENCE: Rubacky, E. P., **"Appearance: Likes and Dislikes,"** *Sensory Evaluation of Appearance of Materials, ASTM STP 545,* American Society for Testing and Materials, 1973, pp. 154-184.

ABSTRACT: The importance of any consensus of people's likes and dislikes, and the practical value thereof, are often obtunded by the large variances of human hedonic behavior within and between people. Means to cope with these problems by the handling of such data, and means by which to constrain the magnitude via suitably high speed data collection systems are reviewed. An historical case is cited to show the sensitivity of people's likes and dislikes versus concentration changes, and it is argued that hedonics does not conform with laws of psychophysical intensity for specific or highly focal sensory research. A case is made from broad scope questioning and from actual stimulus work that general human hedonic behavior may or may not agree with that from specific focal studies. A method for classifying such behaviors into nine hedonic types is described together with its application to quantifying changes, or impacts. Visual hedonic data suggest hedonic behavioral patterns exist, are not dependent upon the rating technique, and are essential to analyses or interpretations if a consensus with meaning is to result. Sensory intensity functions, however useful themselves, are deemed inadequate substitutes to measure where hedonic consensus is needed, as well as misleading.

KEY WORDS: senses, perception, behavioral sciences, hedonics

The science of hedonics, simply stated, is the study of likes and dislikes. The ancient Greek roots of the word are "hedonikos" and "hedys," meaning, respectively, "pleasure" and "sweet," and the science is not to be confused with the ethic or philosophy, "hedonism," which demands the pursuit of pleasure or the avoidance of displeasure.

Hedonics is a behavioral science, dealing with outward manifestations of inner processes that may be called decisions. This distinction is important at the outset for several reasons. One is the fact that just about all of the 3.5 billion people now on this planet share a common freedom: the right and the ability to decide whether and to what extent they may like or dislike anything. That means any product, service, issue, idea, attribute, characteristic, performance, or even

[1] President, ASK, formerly Assess Inc., Bethesda, Md., 20014.

another being. Secondly, the freedom to decide notwithstanding, the behavior may or may not correspond with the actual decision for such reasons as politeness or privacy.

The scope of hedonics is obviously rather broad; it is likewise clear that its interactive nature stems not only from the stimuli-response moiety, but also from the behavioral pattern moiety. Psychophysical behavior, on the other hand, can measure loudness, sweetness, brightness, and the like as a function of decibels, sugar concentration, or candellos generally independent of participant patterns of behavior. In other words, sweet-sweeter-sweetest, etc., is primarily perceptual, and conforms to predictable mathematical formulae, whereas individuals know if the sound, the coffee, or the lights are "just right" for reasons beyond sensory acuity and formulae as yet unknown.

Unlike psychophysics again, hedonics must confront style, fashion, and vogue. Its breadth, therefore, extends to social rather than merely personal conditions and circumstances. In this respect, stimulus-response may be considered cyclic, replete with "feedback loops," instead of directional in nature. Moreover, it is difficult if not impossible to isolate the roles of the several senses and their stored data (memory, pure or sentient or both) in hedonics. As ordinary as simple eating may be to many people, for instance, it can and does draw upon most of the senses and the memory in hedonic decisions. This does not deny the focal nature of one or more senses, however. Accordingly, it is possible and practical to investigate the hedonics of odor or, indeed, of appearance, the subject of this symposium.

Regrettably, the question of whether or not an "appearance" is pleasing depends for its answer on the inherent properties of the material or product itself and the personal plus social behavioral milieu which prevails or applies. Perforce, it becomes important to know if respondents think of a given tumbler as half-full or half-empty, or even their views on truth-falsity and perception-deception. Is the artificial grass in stadiums the same in appearance to the player and the fan? Are false teeth, bosoms and eyelashes, contact lenses, wigs and toupees, cosmetics in general, tailoring, or ersatz building/decorating materials all deceptions? Can packaging be suitably attractive for merchandising without being fraudulent for buyers? The U.S. Truth in Packaging Law, requiring disclosures about contents, paradoxically protects a public that spends billions on deceptive items to wear while at the market. Point of view thus joins need among the complex factors of hedonics in consumption. One can need, dislike, and still buy; another can like, not need, and buy or not buy. More money than is absolutely essential to warmth and mobility is spent on fur coats and prestige cars, conforming to the Doctrine of Conspicuous Consumption [*1*] [2] without which life can be apathetic and dull.

Likes and dislikes are perplexing. This is especially true in marketing.

[2] The italic numbers in brackets refer to the list of references appended to this paper.

Considering the advance time for production as well as the often-heavy investments behind widely distributed or costly items or both, it is no wonder that producers must have measures of probable consumer reactions to justify their decisions. Rejections may be more important than acceptances to manufacturers, if the costly examples of a post World War II car and a recent shoe material are remembered. In most cases, however, failures are not as well publicized. New-product consultant, Ted Angelus, is quoted [*2*] as saying: "something is wrong in the analysis and design of many product tests when 90% of the consumer products that fail in the U.S. have successful test results." If his data are only reasonably accurate, perhaps more and better hedonic research would be helpful and economically valuable.

This paper will attempt to document the present status of hedonics, some of the pitfalls recognized during six years of such investigations, and some advances which have been made to date in handling problems. It will be necessary to deal with general hedonics first, in order to treat the topic of appearance: likes and dislikes.

History

So far as can be determined, the first recorded scientific study in hedonics was by Fechner [*3*], the famous psychophysicist. He reported on the most attractive proportion between width and height of vertical rectangles, in effect starting with our topic, appearance. Publication dates during the century since Fechner reveal, however, periods of inactivity far longer than the aggregate of years spent on scientific research in hedonics. The result has been an inabundant, general, and specific hedonic literature. Beebe-Center's textbook on pleasantness [*4*] is perhaps an ideal reference that reviews many of the contributions over the years. Systematic searching of the literature will reveal a few hundred publications on the subject, at best. Compared, for example, with a daily volume of some 500 papers on the physiology of the adrenal cortex alone, the void in hedonics is both relative and absolute.

Exception will be taken to the foregoing, but the explanation may lie in search criteria. Neither animal studies nor human forced-choice preference work are included in the context of hedonics. The justification for this is complex. First, liking or disliking is not dependent upon paired or set-comparison stimuli; indeed, the single stimulus technique is recommended generally and is essential in first-time evaluations of anything. Secondly, there is no freedom in forced-choice experiments, especially if between two evils, where a selection does not connote liking. Thirdly, hedonics is complex enough without the inclusion of "forces" (appetitive, sexual, tropistic, etc.), widely regarded as operating in animal behavior, and without the problems of communications from animals. Lastly, there are numerous other reasons, some of which will be discussed later.

The dearth of published material does not suggest that scientific research has not been conducted. Commercial firms might logically be reticent about disclosures of their data if competitive advantage would suffer, although it is also probable that, with the passage of time, little would be lost and much would be gained from revealing outdated findings. Another common example resides in the opinion polls on issues and politicians which find their outlets as magazine and newspaper summaries. In light of established procedural delays in the scientific literature, such surveys are not to be faulted for more timely exposure.

For the purposes of this presentation, attention is drawn to some selected publications. In 1928, Engel [5] observed that, by quantitative judgments of pleasantness/indifference/unpleasantness versus variable concentrations of solutions that his subjects tasted, hedonic appraisals were very sensitive. As a matter of fact, Engel's data raise doubts in many minds when compared with just-noticeable-difference (JND) taste perceptions of intensity using similar solutions, since his curves indicate greater hedonic sensitivity over specific concentration ranges. In 1971, Moskowitz [6] confirmed experimentally with sweeteners that pleasantness ratings depart from the Power Function [7] for taste intensity. As stated previously, it is common lay knowledge that pleasantness need not increase with subjective-objective increases in intensity, and the significance of this recent study actually lies in the admission by a former student-disciple of Stevens that hedonics does not obey this psychophysical law. Moreover, hedonic attitudes of observers potentially may contribute to explanations of divergent findings between laboratories on accelerations (exponential values) of intensity perceptions. There now seems to be a basis upon which to treat hedonics differently from psychophysics if not also to concede that people somehow know precisely what is "just right."

This gives rise to discussion of subjective quantifications. Perhaps few would argue the ability of people to decide qualitatively whether they like, or dislike, or are indifferent about a given thing. Nor would it be disputed that people have degrees of liking and disliking. The question arises from expressing these degrees in a measurable and meaningful manner. The issue is valid and extends to the roles of semantics as well as to units. Rather than entertain arguments as to the merits of such techniques as Magnitude Estimations, cross-modality, and Category Rating Scales, the latter was chosen for simplicity and practicality. In particular, the 9-Point Hedonic Rating Scale of Peryam and Pilgrim [8] was favored. It did not seem too long or too short, and provided a mid-point of indifference or neutrality as well as an historical record of successful application in food hedonics over a broad range of IQ's. This scale was modified slightly by the assignment of digits 1 through 9 [9] from most positive to most negative for scoring without semantics on grounds that these could subsequently be processed by several mathematical formulae from arithmetic to logarithmic. In effect, a distinction is necessary between a functional data collection rating system and the precise equation for interpreting the meanings. While the "cubit" lacked precise value, there can be no doubt that, within limits, it had meaning. The inch became more precise a measurement, but only because it was a convention having a reference standard of relative and arbitrary nature to back it. The science of hedonics clearly lacks a working convention for quantification, and it is doubtful that progress or communication will be enhanced until one is adopted.

Paradoxically, there are published warnings against hedonic evaluations on grounds that the variances in the measures both within and between people are very large [*10,11*]. Mindful of the quantitative nature of variance, *per se,* such admonitions are curious in the absence of defined or described quanta in hedonics. Yet, these are scientific ratifications of the old adage "One man's meat is another man's poison," and admissions that hedonics is not purely qualitative. Equally paradoxical is the use of other distribution and distribution-free statistical methods on hedonic data. So far as can be determined, the literature is devoid of validations of specific applications of parametric and nonparametric statistical routines to hedonic data. For example, conventional means are calculated without first establishing the validity of summating the likes of some people with the dislikes of others. Are apples and oranges able to be added without getting fruit salad?

It is generally agreed upon in subjective research that people use scales quite differently. It is argued, however, that this signals the deficiencies of scales, almost without assent to the possibility that this is an important behavioral trait to observe and monitor. Ratio estimation could inherently obtund or mask recognition of behavioral differences. Furthermore, a very basic question is raised: to what extent can one process hedonic data from an individual and from an aggregate of individuals by the same methods? As a matter of fact, one might also ask if data depicting a person's overall, general hedonic behavior spectrum should receive the same treatment as for a specific focal sensory spectrum, such as appearance or odor likes and dislikes.

Despite the problems and the evident state of hedonic science, its prospects for the future may not be dismal. Committee E-18 on Sensory Evaluation of Materials and Products of the American Society for Testing and Materials this year approved an applied method of hedonic appraisal for institutional foods and beverages, and for several years has had an active Task Group on hedonics. In its first three Special Technical Publications, Committee E-18 barely mentioned this subject and, yet, specifically cited "like and dislike" as 2 of only 5 dimensions of any sensation [*12*]. It is acknowledged that even temporary relief, in the form of practical methods, can and must be provided in the face of rising demands which characterize our present Era of Consumerism. Evidently both producers and consumers have interest in manifest likes and dislikes. Committee E-18 will continue to work on basic and applied hedonics.

In the subsequent section, a quick review will be made of some personal attempts to address problems ranging from data collection to processing in both general hedonics and appearance.

Methods

Figure 1 shows the modified Peryam-Pilgrim Hedonic Rating Scale [*8*]. Positive values are at the left, and negative values at the right. To avoid semantics, the user is instructed to apply the term, from among the samples shown, which is deemed most appropriate for each question. Note that the Scale has a "V" form, rather than its original linear configuration, and that the numbers opposite each other add, in pairs, to 10 with the exception of the lone "neutral" value of 5. All scoring is restricted to the use of these single digits, and in some special cases, the number 0 (zero) is added to permit distinctions between "No Opinion" (ignorance) and a "neutral" or "indifferent" response. The zero is especially useful in questioning sessions, but is not permitted with actual stimuli. Subjects find the scale easy to learn and to use, although it has been suggested that the numbering should be reversed, that is, with 9 as the most positive score. In work with children, the numbers can be replaced by smiles and frowns reflecting the degrees.

While the scale is useful in field conditions necessitating manual entries, a technique was developed for remote keypunching of scores into data cards, as

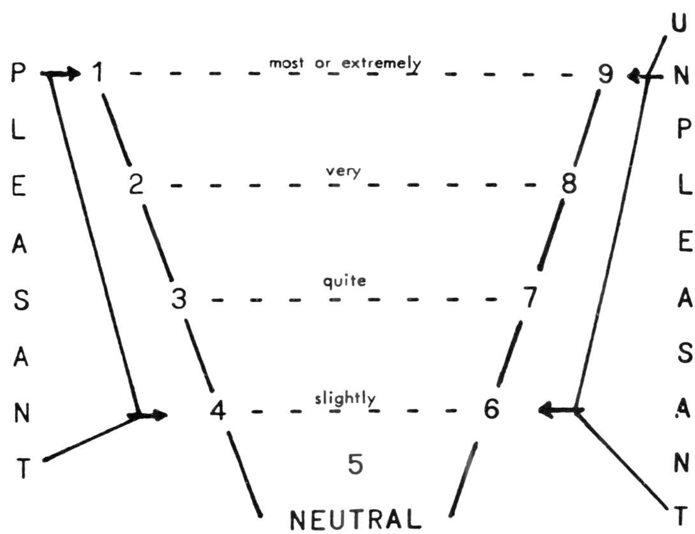

FIG. 1–*Hedonic rating scale* [8]; *users instructed to select appropriate positive or negative terms such as like-dislike, agree-disagree, for-against, favor-oppose, accept-reject and others.*

described in the appended reprint [*13*]. In brief, this semiautomatic technique is feasible via a push-button console for up to five respondents at a time; each merely presses the appropriately numbered (or smiled/frowned) button to enter a score. By virtue of a time-delay feature, a score can be changed, and two buttons cannot be depressed simultaneously to avoid double-punching. The keypunch (SRP) is fed by a monitor and is under the control of a stepper unit (SU) which takes care of automatic sequencing of card columns and the entry of fixed or semi-fixed data. While a recent modification permits real time to be automatically recorded, the monitor must enter lapsed times, and also has options to enter up to six other variables according to experimental needs. In operation, the limits of this configuration are from 4 to 5 stimuli or questions per minute to from 1 to 5 respondents, or about 20 to 25 data points (dp) per minute. It is also hard-wired to the booths, limiting collection to a few yards distance.

Figure 2 shows schematically the components of a fully-automatic system which is now operational. Scores may be entered via telephone, orally for the dial type or by button in the tone type, using the same scale. Data are collected in three ways: on a tape-recorder (B_2); remote activation of a keypunch (E); or directly into a computer (F_2). This updated system utilizes equipment that can be bought or leased, and is generally available rather than unique. It extends the distances over which hedonic data can be entered only to the limits of telephone services. A single respondent can enter 10 scores per minute, or more, depending upon alloted post-stimuli intervals thereby increasing the rate as well as the distance. Contrary to belief, the system can test both questions and stimuli for reactions, but the latter requires special facilities. Practically, the collection and processing of data of this kind usually does not warrant on-line, real-time capability, but it is possible without modification of design. Through a service firm, access to this is currently feasible via a toll-free (namely, an 800 number) line callable from any phone anywhere in the nation, or by an entire network such as the Federal Telephone System (FTS). While presently overdesigned, there is no computer cost if access is not made, and almost simultaneous coverage of people's hedonic views can be achieved from many parts of the country.

While advantage is taken of existing communication and computer hardware, it is the software, or programs for handling the data that also have importance. The computer programs are modular in design. Source, or raw, scoring data are kept by individual, regardless of time, day, or frequency. When processing begins, these data are stored in the memory unit, unscrambled for listings, and subjected to production of basic result statistics. This output is then optionally subjected to various tests of significance, distributions, and goodness-of-fit. In this manner, a number of experimental designs can be employed without necessitating special programs each time. Formatting of statistical analyses

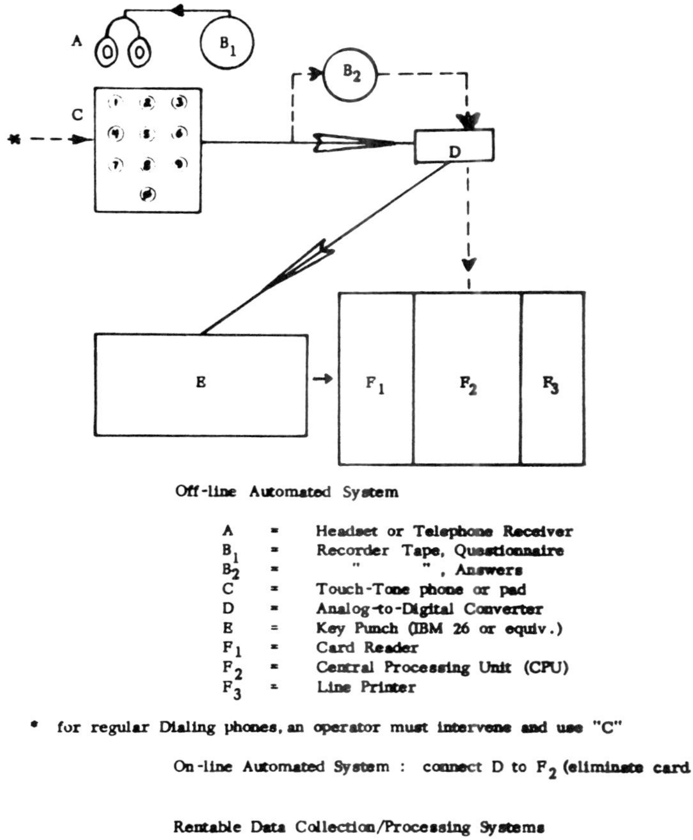

FIG. 2–*Schematic components of a fully-automated system.*

permits the election of one or all available statistical routines on command; where special design features are indicated or required, these can be quickly introduced into the primary module. The two-stage approach trades off the advantage of uninterrupted flow from input to output with the speed of experimental design since the latter could incur delays in writing, editing, compiling, storing, and proving with each program. Regardless of the design variables, the first stage produces such result statistics as: averages (means, medians, and modes), absolute and percentile incidences, and variance functions (sums, sums of squares, and standard deviations).

Among the processing routines developed for hedonic data, the basic one entails a departure from the Aggregate Judge Method (AJM) in which the scores of all respondents to a given stimulus or question are summed to yield a mean response for the group. Rather, the Individual Judge Method (IJM) is used. In brief, this treats all scores by an individual first to yield an hedonic response pattern. Functions of these patterns are then taken from all respondents to yield an hedonic consensus. It is to be noted that this requires multiple responses by all respondents, but also permits a defined group to be treated as if it were an individual so long as all participating respondents remain throughout such studies. In this regard, the IJM allows anonymity of people in a given group. The IJM invokes certain terminology, familiarity with which bears upon the subsequent results in this paper. Prior to explaining these terms, it is to be noted that when this was originally presented [*14*], it was proposed as a convention since, in its pooled form, it could handle scoring by Category Scales, Magnitude Estimation, and Ratio Estimation (although the Shift Factoring form applied only to the former).

There are four terms used in this method: they are the Slopes, Tones, Shifts, and Impacts. The latter two (Shifts and Impacts) are respective changes in the first two. The Slopes are geometric concepts of the relationships; the NP Slope expresses this relationship for scores Neutral and Pleasant, while the NU Slope applies to the one for scores Neutral and Unpleasant. The Hedonic Tone (HT) is the algebraic net of the NP and NU Slopes. These are derived as shown in Table 1.

A graphic display of these slopes may be seen in Fig. 3.

Let the foregoing reflect a "Before" status; then similar processing of "After" status data would yield new Slopes and a new Tone. Without doing actual calculations, both sets of these can be graphically displayed, as shown in Fig. 4 (note arrows). Attention is drawn to the fact that both Before and After Slopes have changed. But, these Shifts are not of equal magnitude on both sides. Because respondents are not forced to any decision, it is not essential that a

TABLE 1–*The Pooled method.*

Actual ratings by each individual, or collectively for a group, are processed to yield both graphic and derived value displays. The steps are as follows:

1.	scores	1	2	3	4	5	6	7	8	9	total
	frequency raw	0	0	0	3	6	5	7	3	1	25
	pooled f			3		6		16			25
	pooled, %			12		24		64			100

2. determine NP = different % (P – N) = 12 – 24 = –12 = –12 divided by k = –12/40 = –.300
3. repeat above for NU = different % (N – U) = –40; –40/40 = –1.000
4. determine HT = algebraic net of NP and NU = –.300 + –1.000 = –1.300

NOTE–k, the constant 40 above is arbitrary; its selection was based upon both the Pooled and Shift Factoring forms.

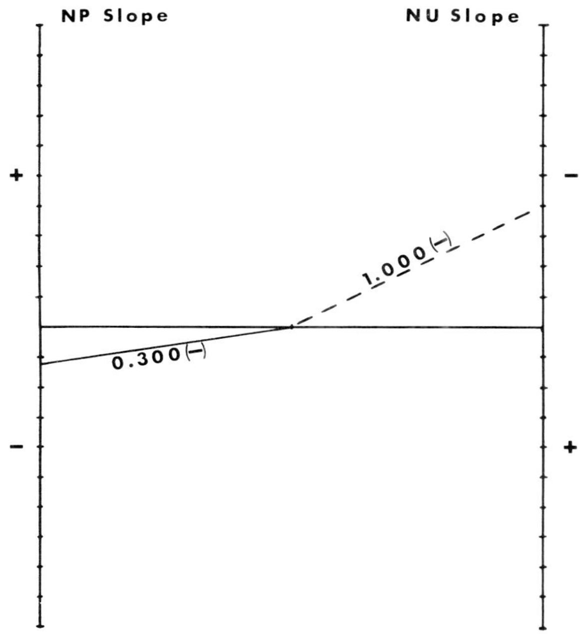

FIG. 3–*Graphic display of the hedonic slopes.*

change on one side be reflected on the other due to the option of "neutral" or "indifferent." Behaviorally, this, in fact, occurs at times, while at other times scores move up or down the scale in degree without altered qualitative changes.

Retrospective review of substantial hedonic data from many individuals, responding to questions (many and varied) and to stimuli by this technique disclosed behavioral patterns, or "ways" of reacting. By invoking a semaphore-like system of oblique and horizontal NP and NU "arms," a classifying technique evolved by which these patterns fit into nine types. People and things (products, etc.) could be classified as a result. This is shown in Fig. 5.

Once again arbitrarily, slopes with values ±0.200 were made horizontal, and all others oblique at 45 deg from the vertical axis, with solid lines on the NP side, and dotted lines on the NU side. Using whole percentages only, there are 5050 possible slope-value combinations which are reduced to nine types in all. The number of combinations per type is finite yet not the same for each. If the arbitrary value of ±0.200 is increased or decreased, this alters the number of combinations per type, but does not yield equal possibilities, mathematically. There is no implication that these combinations per type reflect the incidences among people or things. That is, the fact of 96 ways in 5050 to yield Type V,

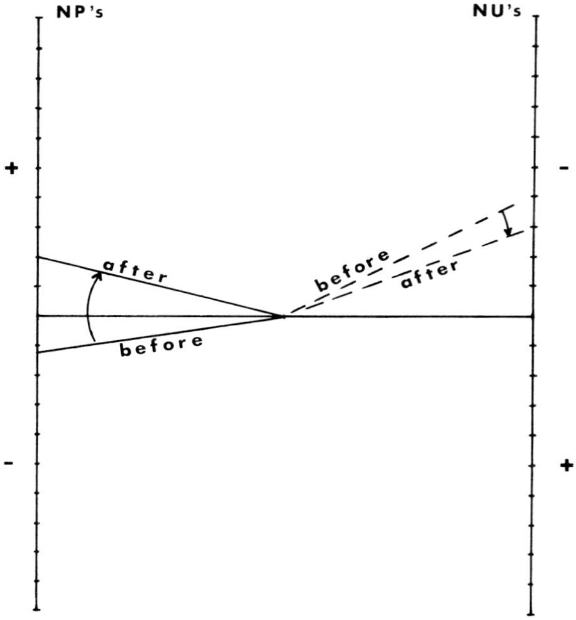

FIG. 4–*Graphic display of unequal changes in the two hedonic slopes.*

for example, does not signify that this is the ratio of Type V people anywhere, although it may occur.

The practical value of these types lies in the readiness of detecting very significant changes, a sort of "screening." If two sets of hedonic data reveal (*a*) any diagonal type change except for V's relative to the corner types (I's, III's, VII's, and IX's), or (*b*) any double-jump horizontally or vertically, then one can immediately suspect high significance. It is possible that other changes may be significant, such as within a given type, as well as between adjacent cells, but these should be more cautiously examined as a routine. A border-line III can, with slight change, become a II, a V, a VI, or even another III without significance. For these reasons, it is suggested that one first become familiar with graphic displays, which are conceptual. In time, one will do this mentally and depend more upon actual Slope and Tone values.

To ascertain hedonic effects on a panel or a populace, the Shifts and Impacts can be tabulated, summarized, cross-footed to verify entries, and averaged. This is shown in Table 2.

Examination of this summary consensus reveals that ten judges freely and, almost in a uniquely individualistic manner, responded. Their actual raw scores are reflected in these transformations. There is no way, from these values, to

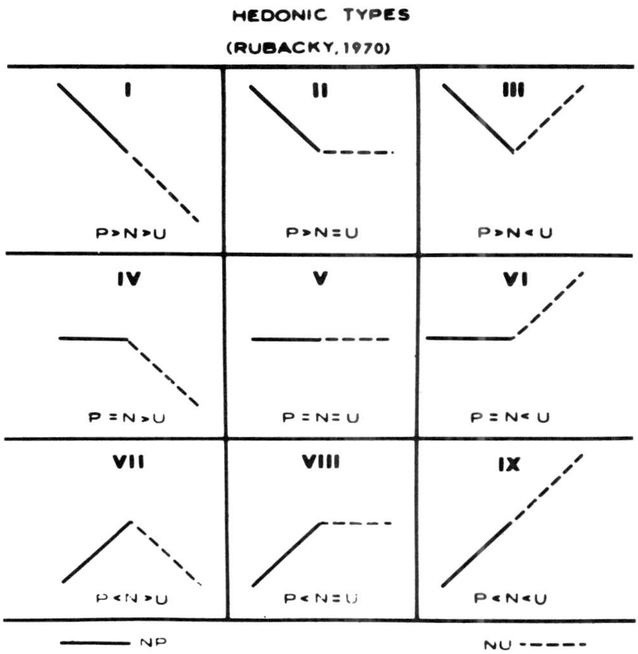

FIG. 5–*The nine hedonic types of people or things.*

TABLE 2–*Hedonic impact–consensus–summarized effects on all judges.*

Judge #	NP Shift	NU Shift	Impact
1	1.100 +	0.625 +	1.725 +
2	0.250 +	1.000 +	1.250 +
3	...	0.150 +	0.150 +
4	0.125 –	0.900 +	0.775 +
5	0.800 +	0.800 –	...
6	0.775 +	0.050 +	0.825 +
7	1.250 +	0.975 –	0.275 +
8	0.075 +	0.150 –	0.075 –
9	0.675 +	0.775 +	1.450 +
10	0.550 +	0.550 –	...
Algebraic Sums	5.350 +	1.025 +	6.375 +
Means	0.535 +	0.102 +	0.638 +

Diagnosis–A slight positive consensus due primarily to increased pleasantness and no decreased unpleasantness of note[*9*].

deduce what types of individuals participated. Judge 5, for example, reveals both increased pleasantness and increased unpleasantness. How? These are data from a study on the hedonic effectiveness in mouth odors, before and after using a breath-freshening product. For some, the effect was improvement while for others it was the reverse—indicating the interaction of the product with the users. Quantitatively, Judge 5 ended with no net Impact, which was not the case with other judges except 10. A final point is that when dealing with changes, as opposed to actual ratings or first applying the AJM, one can isolate the variances due to the respondents and the agent. This, of course, bears upon the recognition of significance in statistical tests. It is submitted that this is a technique for handling hedonic ratings that truly reflects what happened while providing sensitivity that is obscured if scores are aggregated (and potentially cancelled out as changes). Those with hedonic data may wish to try this in comparison to other processing results. The tedium of the Pooled technique, of course, is eased by computers.

Another treatment of hedonic data which may be of interest is the Litchfield-Wilcoxon Method [*15*] which is an all-or-none rather than a graded response technique. It is widely applied in pharmacology and toxicology, and plots incidence as percentage versus given dose levels using a logarithmic/probability-unit coordinates. In hedonics one can pick a criterion, such as percent P, percent U, or percent (P+N) and percent (U+N) versus a quantitative increment (loudness, concentration of ingredient, etc.). Figure 6 displays a case example.

It will be noted in Fig. 6 that a stray point appears to the right of the curve. In this didactic example, it reflects a consensus decline in percent P as the ppm's continued to increase. This is to illustrate the fact that another criterion, such as the percent U can likewise be plotted to yield a curve which, when evaluated versus the percent P results, provides a simple basis for "optimization." This term refers to the level at which the optimum hedonic effectiveness is attained. If, for instance, a single product is all that can be made, the optimization point is that at which any greater increase, or lesser amount, will not please as many people or as much. It can be applied to preparing a meal for soldiers on a given base, or to a civic project, or even to a product for use in a special region and by a special group of users.

Though somewhat terse, these are the methods of collecting and processing hedonic data which have been in use over the past six years. Through the use of automation in communications and computer technology, it has been possible to conduct general studies and particular focal sensory hedonic experiments in the knowledge that results may easily be subjected to numerous analytical tests. The flexibility that this affords, especially with hundreds of thousands of ratings compares favorably with the ability afforded in varying factors of experimental design. The real test of any method, however, is its use by peers.

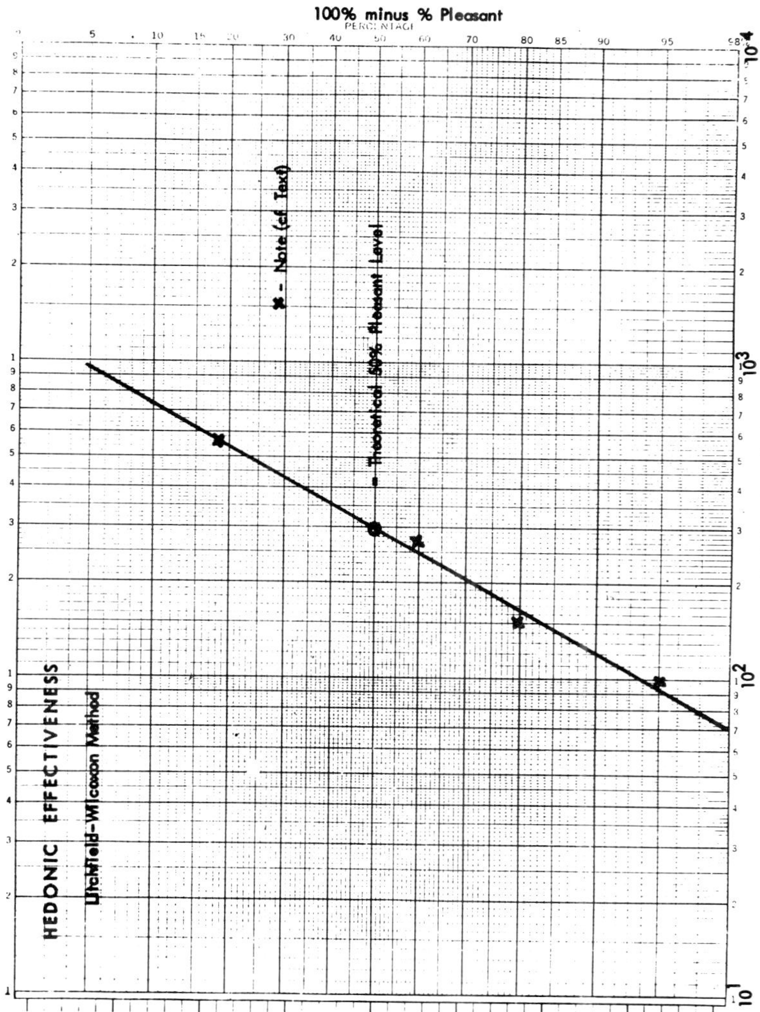

FIG. 6–A *product optimization curve using percent P data; to be analyzed in conjunction with similar curves using other percent data.*

Results

Figure 7*a* shows the frequency distribution curves of the Conklin studies[*16*] of 1923, using the six issues by two scales on 1699 college students. The same results are shown in Figure 7*b*, using the Slopes from the Pooled technique. Notwithstanding the author's conclusion that the two scales explain the apparent differences in the curves, the hedonic responses of the students show no difference in this re-plotting (save for a slight one in the NU Slopes) or in their actual views. The fact is that none of the students was able to use either the 9 or the 13-point scales fully, with only six issues to score. Moreover, it is to be expected that any scale from 3 to 21 points would yield its own, unique frequency-distribution curve. That is not the point of the study; rather, it was to determine whether different size scales would affect the hedonic judgments.

Figure 8 shows the distinction between psychophysical intensity and hedonic appraisal results. Where the lower curve "breaks" could be considered the optimization in this example. In essence, this is the kind of result which Moskowitz[*6*] found for sweetners. The upper, dotted curve indicates the 1:1 relationship between perceived and actual changes in intensities. It is noteworthy, because sight and sound would have curves above this line, being termed "positively accelerated." This refers to the fact that perceptions are made with slight changes in intensity. "Negatively accelerated" functions obtain for smell, taste, and touch. They would be found under the dotted curve, since large changes are needed for perceptions of intensity. This must be kept in mind when doing hedonic appraisals in general, but are most important in focal sensory evaluations where hedonics may be appearance or odor or a similar concern (heavily or solely dependent upon a given sense). Since most people eat, and assuming that intensity influences all hedonic ratings, the perceptions of the various senses are probably contributing to varying extents from the time the eye sees, the ear hears, the nose smells, and the mouth feels and tastes a bite of steak, a potato chip, or a sip of a beverage.

Despite the view that hedonics is fraught with variance problems between and within individuals rating things, the question should really be: how accurate or precise are hedonic ratings? As an indication, Figs. 9*a* and 9*b* from Engel's[*5*] work are shown. At the top is quinine sulfate, and at the bottom is cane sugar. Portions of both figures indicate or suggest, if they do not prove, that rather small concentration differences are hedonically perceived. Yet, the bitter and the sweet (both taste functions primarily) yield diverse plots when incidences of ratings are matched with concentrations. Engel did many solutions, and this is true of most all the curves.

In 1971, results were published[*17*] in which a small group of volunteers responded to questionnaires (Q's) given on 20 occasions in one year. The hedonic scoring and data processing were as previously described. There were 50 questions (q's) or items in each Q, with some q's repeated from time to time.

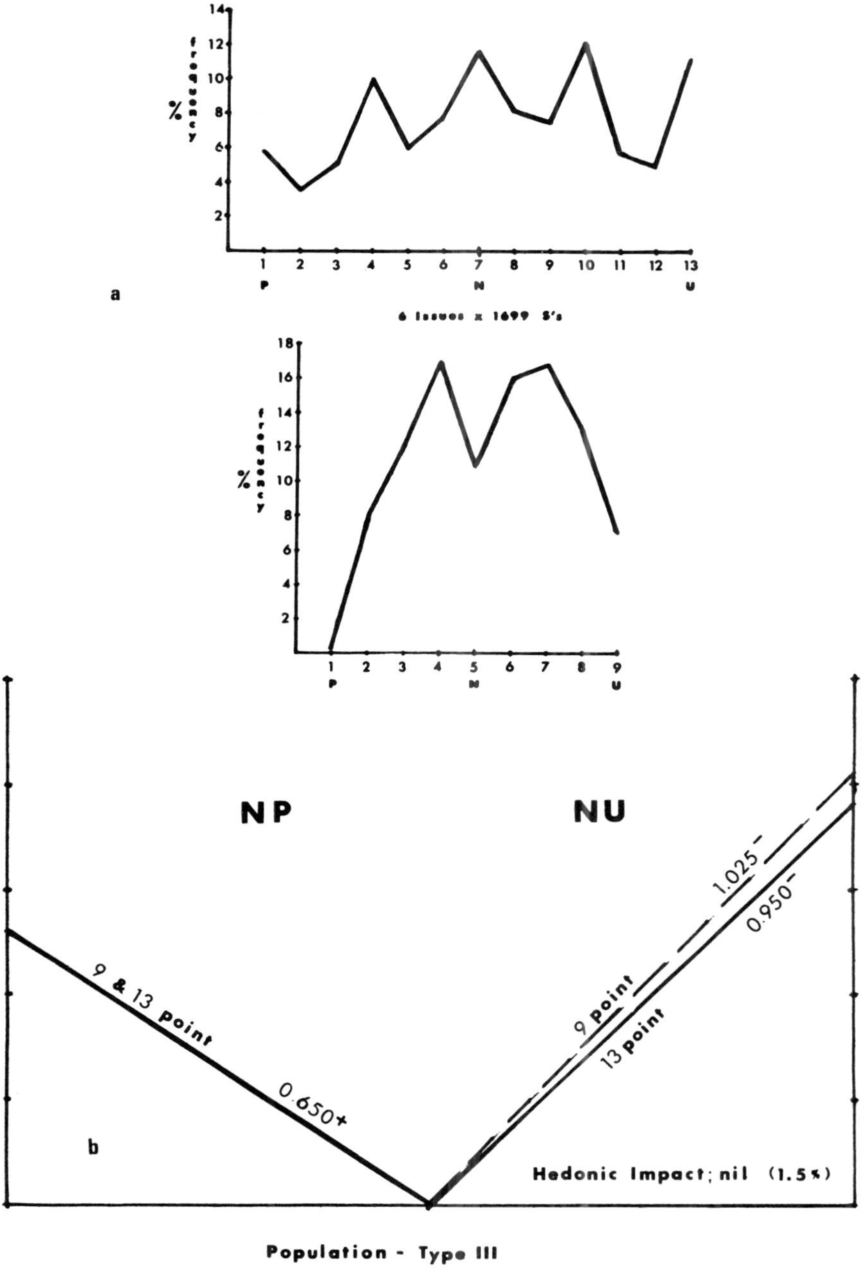

FIG. 7–(a) *Conklin's*[16] *frequency distribution curves of rating scores from 1699 subjects on 6 issues using a 13-point* (*top*) *and then a 9-point* (*bottom*) *hedonic rating scale 3 months later.* (b) *The same results shown as hedonic slopes using the pooled method.*

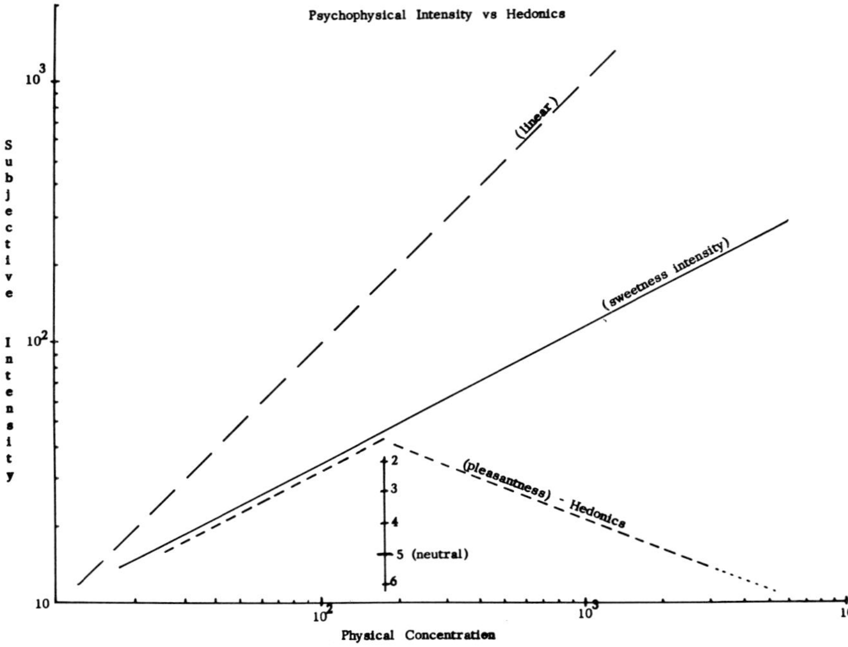

FIG. 8–*Psychophysical intensity versus hedonics.*

The latter enabled repositioning of items to check for proximity and contrast and similar effects. Approximately 10 min time per Q was required. Each respondent provided 1000 hedonic ratings over the four subexperiments of five Q's each. It was found that, in general, the Hedonic Tones from Q to Q and from subexperiment to subexperiment were rather stable. Each person was typed by subexperiment and questionnaire; each item (q) was typed also, often up to five times. Typing of each q was additionally done as a consensus for the subjects (S's). This stability was impressive. What was intriguing about it, however, was the fact that "cross-overs" occured without marked effect on stability. A cross-over is "major" if from one side of the scale to the other, and "minor" if from one side to the middle (or vice versa), and these are flagged by double or single asterisks on the print-outs. In all, over 250 different q's were used in the study, and these encompassed a wide variety of things, from clothing to conditions and ideas. It was concluded that, within limits and in spite of altered hedonic ratings at times, the stability reflected fixation of one's hedonic behavioral pattern. In other words, an hedonic optimist (Types I and II) remains one; an hedonic pessimist (Types VIII and IX) also remains unchanged.

The next study was to have a given group choose any two of the 20 Q's,

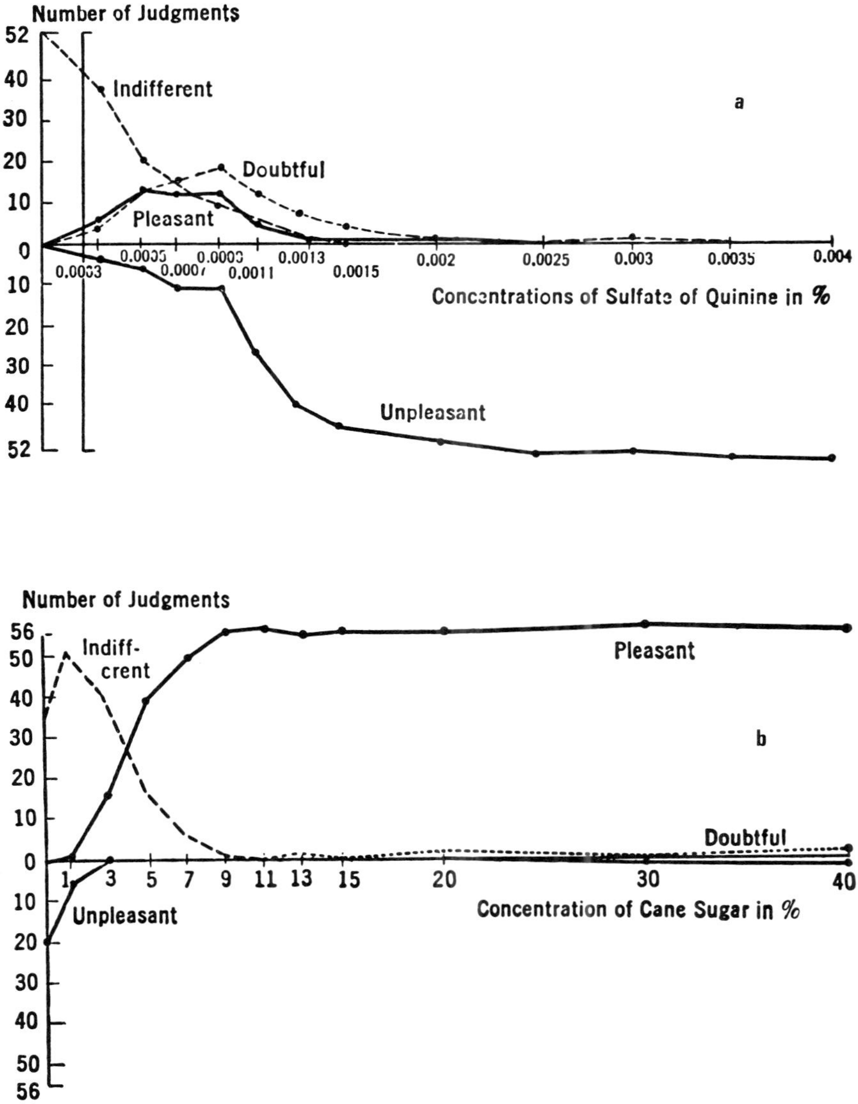

FIG. 9–(a) *Curve representing the hedonic tone of solutions of sulfate of quinine for ten observers in six sittings.* (b) *Similar curve substituting solutions of cane sugar.*

present each with a rest period of ten or more minutes, and process the Slopes/Tones. These same-day tests given in no less than six major cities in the United States confirm the stability of the Hedonic Tones of respondents. A reason for this study was the fact that, during the one year of the prior study, certain instabilities were found, but almost invariably when sizeable, they occured in women. Early in 1972 [*18*], investigations were reported addressing this. First, women 16 years and older were given Q's from among our selection list at six-day intervals. When the Slopes and Tones were processed and plotted, the evidence suggested that each female had a basic type from which a negativity, a positivity, or both were found, corresponding to what could be a reproductive cycle. The few cases of positivity were approximately two weeks away from the negativity. Regardless of the degree of negativity, however, the suggestion was monthly. So as not to prejudice responses and elicit compensatory behaviors, none of the women were told of the intention to evaluate their results versus time or cycles (which were not known, either). Based upon this presumptive evidence, women whose cycles were determined were subjected to spontaneous hedonic questioning without knowing why. Since the frequency was random in their minds, it was not associated so far as is known. Figure 10 shows two cases having noticeable negativity just prior to onset of menses compared with typical base-line Slopes. In the upper, negativity is more marked, and consists of both NP and NU shifts; in the lower case, negativity was less severe, and primarily due to increased unpleasantness. While not proof in the strict sense of the word, these findings suggest that pre-menstrual tension, so widely acknowledged, can be described via hedonic indices. Evidence was insufficient and inconclusive that positivity may coincide with ovulation. Studies planned in this regard include tests of women using anovulatory pills versus controls such as with IUD's and tubal ligations or nothing.

The Hedonic Tones in these women varied from ±2 to ±25 percent, compared with a range of ±3 percent for over 95 percent of all men, and women tested twice on the same day. Since the maximum change, using the formula above for the Pooled technique, is 5.000, the most sizable female time changes were of the order of 1.250. The q's employed in these tests were the same for men and women, and the stabilities of these items also deserves mention. Where replicate data exist, from 2 to 5 times per q, for about 10 percent of the 250-odd q's, there was no evidence of sex-related trends despite the fact that total "cross-overs" ranged from 2 to 33 percent. Hence, both stability and lability were noted for various q's. A major contribution to lability was found to be proximity rather than position, *per se.* The word, "exhaustion" typifies this. A deliberate positioning after the term, "orgasm," yielded a far more positive Hedonic Tone overall than from any other proximity. The Q's require less than 10 min time apiece, but "exhaustion" did not show significant change when positioned early to late in a given questionnaire. Moreover, near duplications of

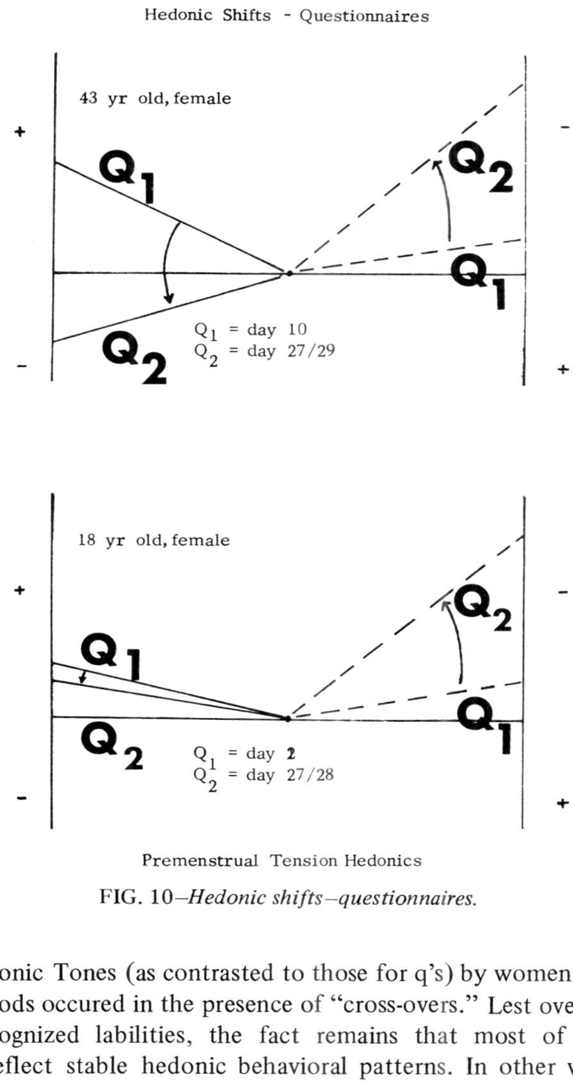

FIG. 10–*Hedonic shifts–questionnaires.*

personal Hedonic Tones (as contrasted to those for q's) by women over much of the time periods occured in the presence of "cross-overs." Lest over-emphasis be given to recognized labilities, the fact remains that most of the data for individuals reflect stable hedonic behavioral patterns. In other words, people tend to remain as typed, not the reverse, whether more pessimistic or more optimistic in expressing likes and dislikes.

In another experiment, 22 adults were given color stimuli using an automated slide projector with set on-off intervals and without assigned context for any colors. In this study, no scalar categories were prescribed, and ratings were made along a line with extremely pleasant at one end, the opposite at the other end, and a midpoint for neutral or indifferent ratings. Subjects were instructed only to make a mark along each line following presentation of the color slide. The same S's were previously and subsequently given Q's for ratings via the 9-Point Category Rating Scale for comparison of these visual data to general hedonics. For incidences in the visual study, the number of marks, regardless of how near or far from the poles or midpoint, were counted as P, N, and U ratings so that Slopes and Tones could be determined. There were several interesting results in these experiments, but the two main ones were (1) the patterns of marking along the lines in the visual part, and (2) the lack of a firm relationship between general and focal visual responses. There were numerous instances of replicate slides, and cross-overs occured often and extensively for all S's. The Appendix shows some examples of marking patterns of some select S's, corresponding to extreme polarity for all slides, centering tendency, and general or random marking all along the lines. This pseudo form of Magnitude Estimation reveals patterns hitherto attributed to scale properties believed inherent with categorizing, independent of the number of points available for use. A second finding was that some S's yielded quite similar to quite different behaviors, on the basis of patterns of the Slopes. In short, the general hedonic behavior for the questionnaires did not necessarily equate to that of the visual hedonics even though, at times, this did occur with remarkable uniformity between tests. A person could thus be a Type III for the Q's and the color stimuli, or two distinct types which are not even close, or anywhere in between such results.

In May of 1969, Committee E-18 had 57 of its members participate in a demonstration done by one of the Task Groups within its ranks. The theme of this project was to illustrate the role of isolating a specific sense. In physiology and medicine, the functions of organs are often studied by temporary or permanent removal and comparisons of the "with" and "without" results. Some examples of this demonstration seem pertinent to the theme of this paper. One is to isolate vision in smoking. While the blind may not find the results strange, those who try with a blindfold are often impressed with the fact that when using one's own brand to do the test, it is extremely difficult or disconcerting under these conditions to tell if a given cigarette is lit or unlit when presentations are made randomly by another. The best results are obtained if the smoker has been smoking already during that day and if the brand is not mentholated. Drawing down, or "dragging," and inhaling from the mouth is done for each presentation as is the smoker's custom. Another visual case was the ingestion of so-called crackers-and-cheese while blindfolded. Each presentation permitted smelling, tasting, chewing, and mouth-feel, using only one kind of cracker for all trials. Half the participants assisted those who ingested. The hedonically most positive results did not occur with real cheeses, but with a nontoxic but odoriferous gel-stick sliced to emulate cheese. Other tests included visual-tactile trials with textile materials represented (as for shirts), common sounds without associated visuals, and paint-panels rated visually, by touch, and for sound emissions.

Without exception, all these confirmed the interdependence of the senses operating together, and the loss of ability or confidence following isolation, whether the task was identification or hedonic evaluation. Since those in attendance were experts or specialists in sensory evaluations, these demonstrations served to focus upon a broader view than many might have had from stressing one sense in their work. It was obviously not new, and many were familiar with similar, published studies as with green mashed potatoes and with sherberts flavored and colored in unusual combinations. Such findings as these crystallize the multi-sensory nature of hedonics.

More than 100 adults participated in an experimental survey as to the desirability of color-coding various types of pills and tablets. Respondents were given certain drug classifications, such as for headaches, etc., and were simply asked to specify the color each would like associated with the class. There was no rule against using a color more than once or against colors in combination, and the inference was made that a system was being contemplated rather than mere coding by color for some drugs only. Most interesting was the inclusion of "blues" by so many people. Decades ago, when mercury compounds were used in the treatment of syphillis, the Guy's Hospital Blue Pills were socially tell-tale in nature. The stigma affected the drug industry, and this color was avoided. Among thousands of marketed drugs today, blue is still rarely used, even though antibiotics have since replaced mercurials. Other results ensued from this study, but this finding is singled out to illustrate the effects of time on people, and the orientation or prejudice within an industry—a subpopulation of the overall public—in hedonics. Moreover, customary use of color, such as white for aspirin-containing drugs, will make changes difficult, and blues will probably be introduced slowly in the future.

In the past six years, a considerable amount of our work has entailed hedonics of mouth-odor including measures of effectiveness of mouthwashes. Generally, 25 S's receive an initial rating, after which a product is used, and subsequent ratings are made at intervals post-use by special odor judge panels. The S's have, at times, also provided hedonic ratings of the mouthwashes overall, for taste-flavor, and for mouth-feel. One such study was done in which the product was tried in two forms: colored as usual and colorless. Despite no other difference, the S's clearly were more negative about the colorless form on these indices. Appearance affected the results.

TRANSPO '72, the First U.S. International Transportation Exposition, was an occasion, covering 9 days on-site and an additional 30 days for follow-up, for extensive application of these hedonic methods. The contractor (Bourgeois Science Services, Ltd.) used manual, semi and fully-automatic systems to appraise over 100 features of this Exposition hedonically. Some 2000 people from among the general public, visiting scientists and engineers, and exhibitors provided hedonic ratings covering operational, educational, and entertainment aspects, as well as economic values and future Transpo's. While a full report has been made to the Government, several highlights bearing upon the general and the appearance aspects of hedonics are cited here (with permission).

(Note: this portion has been revised appreciably due to the fact that the color photos depicting results and concepts require both special printing and extensive explanation, even more so in black-and-white.)

Among features evaluated, there were overall and first impressions, the Theme Area, the aerial shows, cleanliness and general condition (washrooms, toilets, litter), mobility modes (past, present, and futuristic), and exhibits to cite some examples.

Comparisons of results were made between groups of people and as a function of time on-site or conditions (before-after). Nearly 35 000 hedonic ratings were obtained, and people found the scale to be simple. Only from 2 to 5 min were needed per person, in itself appealing. While not sought, acclaim was given to the search for both positive and negative hedonic responses by the people. System speed afforded results to administrators of Transpo '72 on a same-day basis. The telephonic capability enabled the 371 exhibitors to respond anonymously from all over the nation (plus Canada) with candor and on the basis of 30 days time to allow actual results comparison with on-site impressions.

By the end of the first day, public ratings on litter and trash showed decline in hedonic Tones with time; promptly, a supplementary collection contract was issued, with subsequent day's ratings of this index corroborating the decision even when attendance was much greater. The toilets and washrooms yielded hedonic ratings that declined with peak crowds at 5 percent per hour. Service personnel were ample in numbers, but differential studies pointed out that the hedonics were more affected by the interiors of the portable units than the waiting lines or the odors emitted from the service ports (externally accessible). Broken light bulbs, cleanliness, and paper supplies were pin-pointed from rating data; units were locked up and taken out of use. The management reassigned personnel with stress upon interior service during peak attendance (late morning till late afternoon) commencing with the second day, and ratings by the people returned to initial approval levels. The practical value of heeding public hedonics by proper application of resources with conditions was clear, and extra staff costs were not incurred needlessly. The aerial shows could be viewed both from the general site and from special stands for an extra fee. Hedonically, ratings indicated that one person in six was indifferent, and one in sixteen was negative about these 2-h shows, held once or twice each day. Despite this, no pictorial evidence was found that either locale produced different hedonic results. The photographs also showed that the shows almost uniformly attracted attention of all those who were outside buildings. Attraction and hedonic appeal evidently are separate phenomena in spectacular appearances. Overall and first impressions were quite favorable, both in the rating data and early newspaper/TV accounts.

Attendance figures began to increase, and by the final weekend reached saturation. This is important because of prevailing local press reports just prior to the Exposition. In brief, they recounted a major traffic jam a few years earlier (with only one fifth the expected Transpo attendance) over the entire 14-mile access highway, and a forecast that it would be "the biggest Federal blunder since Custer" because of doubts that the construction would be finished by opening day. Despite the extensive newspaper, radio, and TV coverage of both of these gloomy forecasts, the hedonic ratings of traffic flow and control were highly (perhaps excessively) positive, with no jams or major delays. What effect this had on the moods of those attending is unknown, but it was probably beneficial. Crowd sizes ranged from 30 to 200 thousand daily, with the largest attendance on the final weekend. In the interim, publicity had shifted to accurate reporting of facts along with acclaim for the Exposition and its management.

Appearance was a major factor, as the name suggests, both in the stimuli to the people (exhibitions) and the people themselves on other people. Expectation in appearance hedonics was probably a most significant factor, as well.

Summary

These brief results have been highlighted to draw attention to several features of hedonics. The first reflects the application of new formulae in processing data from a half-century ago. The second points to differences in psychophysical intensity phenomena and quantitative hedonics. Next, questionnaire studies were cited to signify the typing of people and items hedonically, with indications of behavioral stability and certain labilities in women with respect to cyclic events. Fourthly, using visual stimuli, comparisons were made in behavioral patterns to those observed via questionnaires to indicate that specific focal hedonic studies may or may not correspond with general patterns. After this, the role of isolation of a sense on decisions and confidence was pointed out. Sixth, temporal influence was exemplified via the blue color for pills, and seventh, the affect of conditioning on hedonics was indicated when the mouthwash appearance was altered. Finally, numerous other capabilities, and influences on hedonic ratings, were illustrated in the appearance-oriented Transpo '72 Official Survey [*19*]. This latter might serve to indicate the practicality of high-speed hedonic data collection and processing in applied tasks with sensitivity and accuracy.

Discussion

Our beginnings in hedonic research some six years ago were addressed to measuring subjective effects of drugs and cosmetics alone. From inception, semiautomatic data collection was used because of anticipated demands on volume-time aspects of the experimental data. Within two years, it was apparent that customary statistical procedures were deficient, chiefly in their failure to describe mathematically what was observable in the source, or raw, scores. Serendipity prevailed in that retrospective review of the product test-data required only experimentation with statistical procedures. New routines were compiled on the small computer (IBM 1130), and the modular result-statistic cards were rerun with them, a task likely not to have been done manually or even with a programmable desk calculator. The compelling force was the apparent effects of the drugs and cosmetics, even in the opinions of the users.

In the intervening years, the same previously described methods for handling data have been used and compared with such conventional AJM tests as Chi-squares, "t" tests, intercorrelations, and variance analyses. Applications, besides those just noted, have now been extended into wholly unrelated fields to drug and cosmetic studies. Taste-flavor, political opinion, and personnel studies are some other examples. This is, admittedly, a rather narrow spectrum of applications for what is suggested to be a system of value for hedonics in general, and other specific focal sensory hedonic appraisal work. The value and limits, other than inherent in this system, will, of course, rest with time and use by peers.

With respect to the inherent limits, it is already clear that open-ended hedonic evaluations cannot be performed using this system. Where projections of how much more or less of something, such as an ingredient, would increase the pleasantness is of interest to a producer, this system requires experimental formulations. They must be prepared and tested, whereas open-ended data could be quite useful, especially if based upon experience.

Presently, it is already obvious that tests must be extended to distinguish better the designs of studies using "non-consumer beneficiaries" and "consumers" or "buyers." Such design considerations bear upon the individual versus social hedonics, and introduce the role of the non-buyer on the buyer. A woman may, for example, like a given dress enough to purchase it only to find herself devastated by a comment by someone else; she may continue in her own opinion, but never again wear it. This sort of phenomenon occurs in many situations besides style, fashion, and vogue in clothing, such as in community fine arts, architecture, and "eagleton-like" affairs. One might even say that the pursuasive art, advertising, frequently attempts to establish or adjust the social milieu.

Preliminary data from studies where respondents were alone or isolated in booths compared to groups gathered together indicate both tendencies to depart from patterns and similar scores by proximal people on given items. Thus, designs must contemplate constraints on hedonic freedom where isolation may force or obscure, and assembly may do likewise. A consensus in hedonics should have a label, such as "a composite of isolated appraisals" or "appraised in assembly," along with pertinent conditions.

As with any system using numerical values, as actual ratings or assigned to verbal description choices, another inherent limit exists. This is the Principle of Insufficient Reason. Mathematics validly concludes that *A* is greater than *C* if, indeed, *A* is greater than *B* and *B* is greater than *C*. Hedonically, it is possible that such logic is faulty, save for the numerical values. In paired or set comparisons, *A* may be preferred over *B*, *B* over *C*, and then *C* may beat *A*. Just as it is wrong to deduce that Yale will win over Harvard in football because Yale beat Princeton and Princeton beat Harvard, by this principle it can be wrong logically though not statistically in hedonics. One should recall the children's game of "Paper-Scissors-Rock" and consult with a bookie if any doubt remains as to the existence and operation of this principle in life. In hedonics, the problem lies not with statistics, but with interpretations and the logic.

Customarily, the whole is comprised of its parts. While our Hedonic Tones consist of the algebraic sums of the NP and NU Slopes, as proved by cross-footing, the assumption that a consensus of Tones may be compared as if a consensus of Impacts or vice versa, may not be valid. Tones may be as divergent as extreme types, whereas Impacts may not be. In fact, Fig. 11 shows how four

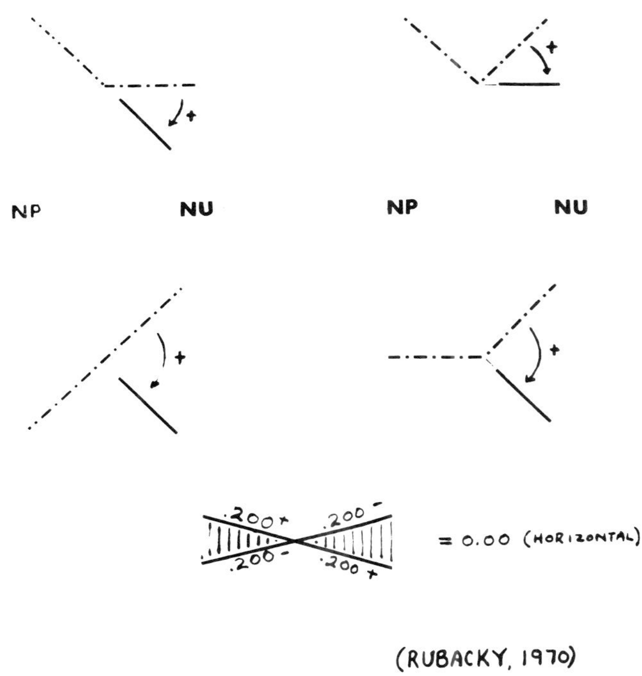

(RUBACKY, 1970)

FIG. 11–*Hedonic impacts in 4 divergent types by similar positive shifts of the NU slopes only* (upper series), *and the slope limits for the horizontals in typing* (lower one).

types (II, III, VI, and IX) all reflect positive Impacts via decreased unpleasantness. The resulting Slopes yield Types I, II, VII, and IV, respectively. It exemplifies why the variances of Impacts are not necessarily as great as with raw scores or Tones.

The keynote of the three concepts (social/individual; the principle; and the sum of the parts/whole) lies not in complexities of this research, since these exist regardless of method or system. Rather, it lies in measuring and knowing what has hitherto been unknown and hence not measured. As in many sciences, the variable may require only identification and measurement while also being uncontrollable. Precisely what the future will provide hedonic science in terms of new or improved formulae and refinements cannot be estimated. Experiments at our laboratory are primarily in two classes: the expansion of scope of applications; and expansion of data processing techniques. One, in addition to the cited Shift Factoring technique, consisted of "weighted" result statistics in which the sort of thing customarily done with academic grades versus course credit loads is being tested. Another is hedonic trend analysis. The advancement of hedonic science will depend, however, upon the contributions of many and a broadening of scope.

Our laboratory and field studies are also aimed at the development of a mathematical model of applied hedonic theory. Tentatively, it is orthogonal; the principal sense invoked is like a pole which is supported by other sensory inputs plus memory (experiences). The final hedonic decision in the model varies with strength of both the pole and the struts. For the present, however, we must establish a hierarchy of the major senses as these participate in subjective judgments of any kind. In terms of appearance, for instance, sight is important, so far as most would think. It can be considered the most distal of the senses, in that stimuli can be received from the greatest distances. Sound would be next-most distal. Smell would come third, and touch would be followed by taste. Yet, assigned importance can resemble a tail swinging a dog. In vision alone one cannot ignore altered acuities, color-blindnesses, astigmatisms, strabismus, and a host of pathologies. To what extent is the hierarchy disturbed by defects in the senses? Does a person rate a steak differently as visual change with age occurs? Can a blind man (functionally or legally) provide appearance ratings in hedonics? Four of our six years of this research was done under the auspices of the Eye Research Foundation of Bethesda, and while proof is insufficient, it would have to be concluded at this stage that hedonic appraisals continue to be made after losses in acuity or blindness. Evidently, changes are usually gradual and the memory contributes markedly in hedonics. The difficulty lies in new and novel experiences, and the sustenance draws from heeding signals via the other senses. If one plots hedonic tones of people by age, and in the absence of extremes of joy and sorrow, there is a general trend to increased negativity as we grow older that may be more significant behaviorally than the acuity of one or more senses, *per se.* In our olfactory acuity work, nearly 500 people have been processed and some 60 have been used by virtue of very high (2 to 5 binary steps over normal) acuity in hedonic work. Taste thresholds for 20 substances have been measured in another 200 people, and in comparative studies low thresholds for taste detections may or may not agree with odor skills. The lesson in multi-sensory research is not the focal skill as much as the total skill. It matters less how a person makes a hedonic decision, as that it is made. An easy experiment is to find someone genetically incapable of tasting phenyl thio-carbamide (PTC) and ask if he or she likes it. The usual result in our hands is no, but only after a few seconds, which is possibly due to perceived smell. They do not realize why, but the response is often rather clear-cut.

Lip-reading is an example of sound having appearance. Compensatory actions by the deaf or near-deaf have, in fact, made it difficult for parents and teachers to recognize children who read lips. Other than intuitive or inborn information, all the rest enters the central nervous system via the senses. Only the rate of stimulation of various senses changes throughout life, the day, or night. It is a continuous process. From an hedonic research viewpoint, the best that can be expected at this stage of the science is to measure the effects under certain conditions and hope to learn. It has been recognized in the drug field that no amount of animal work will ever eliminate actual cautious trials in man. Perhaps in like manner, it will be concluded that no amount of substitute work, whether subjective or objective or both in nature, will eliminate direct hedonic appraisals to determine personal or social or both likes or dislikes.

The Era of Consumerism did not arise without cause. Now, perhaps more than at any prior time in history, there is greater importance in knowing man's likes and dislikes—not just the latter. Communication is massive and rapid, exposing consumers to advocates and champions, whether or not they may be a minority, while also exposing producers to sudden peril or success. Were there meaning for any producer, specifically in the Angelus statement, an inverse correlation could be helpful from lab test to consumer, namely, offer only that which is rejected in the lab. The trouble is that one also needs the results on rejections when tested on consumers to know if this is valid, and to find out how a given new product will correlate for a given new-product maker. Even at 90 percent failure on the market, there is 10 percent remaining that could be wrongly kept off the market by an inverse approach. Rather, it seems that hedonic research must continue.

As a science, hedonics warrants effort and improvement to meet demands. Consumerism has taken away the restaurant and roadside inn experts of yesteryear. In their place is the public, which is unlikely to surrender its new-found, lofty position. They will predictably demand that their likes be retained, their dislikes rectified. Presently, there are substantial and costly programs offered by producers with economic health or survival at stake. In all candor, most of these programs seem negative and therapeutic in nature. If a preventive stage is to be attained, time will probably demand that more positive, diagnostic programs be added or substituted. The "ombundsman," the "recall," the "unconditional guarantee" (of replacement with another, or full refund), the listen-better "hot lines," and the like require action by the consumer, often in the angry state if not also frustrated. It is usually easier to forget it and buy from another in the hope that next time things will improve. Advantage is also taken of this statistically (except in the case of recalls), since it is obvious that most people would not get worked up over smaller purchases any more than some will tell a waiter when service is bad. Hedonics is not at its best with angry or exhilarated people. Producers need to know the views of less polar, more typical people. To do so on a scale fitting their markets is generally believed to be too costly. While that is relative, the real cost must also include the effects of rejection by the public rather than monitoring alone. This must be realistic, and trade-offs are necessary in business.

To summarize, it is felt that this may provide some new ways of measuring hedonic behaviors and some treatments for the data. The overall system is and has been operating, and its speed and scope are presently overdesigned. Cost is not the subject herein, but may be stated as both absolutely and relatively low.

Acknowledgments

The author expresses appreciation to the Eye Research Foundation of Bethesda, Md., Bourgeois Science Services, Ltd., and to C. R. Cavonius for the use of materials herein described. The general assistance of the members of ASTM Committee E-18 Subcommittee 18.02 on Principles of Psychophysical Test Methods is also gratefully acknowledged.

APPENDIX

Following are four photocopies (Figs. 12*a, b, c,* and *d*) of actual scoring sheets from studies of color hedonics using lantern slides. No context was given with each of the 50 stimuli per volunteer human subject. Instructions simply consisted of telling S's to mark along the lines as the stimulus impressed them. Note the examples show that, without a scale but within limits prescribed, there are patterns of scoring. For comparisons with the data from the same S's on questionnaires, using the 9-point Scale, these lines were subdivided into nine parts, and the values at the right indicate the presumed hedonic ratings by such a scale. In some cases, the hedonic types for the color study and the questionnaire work were the same, while in others the S's adopted specific color patterns.

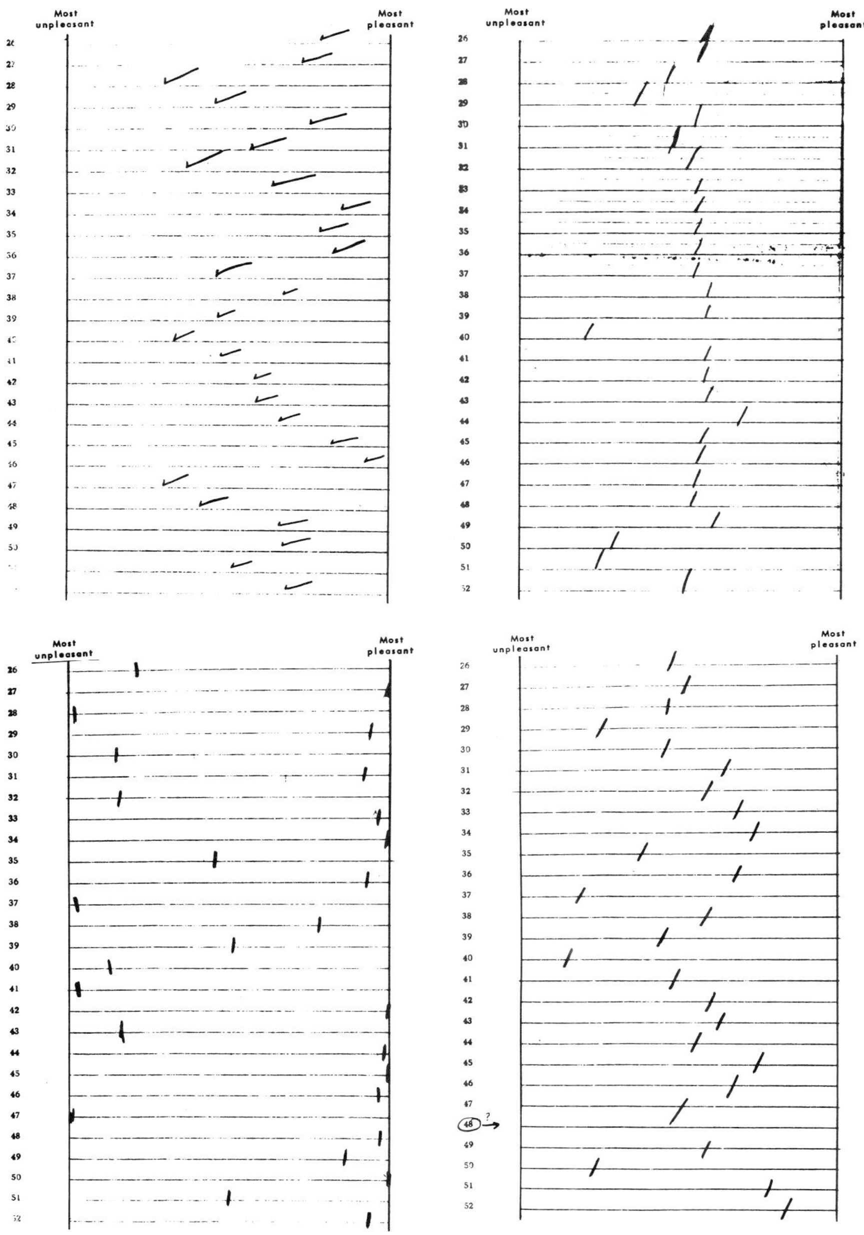

FIG. 12–(a, b, c, and d) *Photocopies of actual scoring sheets from studies of color hedonics using lantern slides; despite the lack of a Category Rating Scale, diverse rating patterns are revealed.*

References

[1] "Doctrine of Conspicuous Consumption," cited by S. Katz of Leber, Katz, and Paccione, New York.

[2] Angelus, Ted, *Business Week,* 4 March 1972, pp. 72-77.

[3] Fechner, G. T., *Vorschule der Aesthetik,* von Breitkopf u. Härtel, Leipzig, 1876.

[4] Beebe-Center, J. G., *The Psychology of Pleasantness and Unpleasantness,* D. Van Nostrand, New York, 1932.

[5] Engel, R., *Archiv Fuer Gesamte Psychologie,* Vol. 44, 1928, pp. 1-36.

[6] Moskowitz, H. R., personal communication, 1971, (subsequently published in *American Journal of Psychology*).

[7] Stevens, S. S., *American Scientist,* Vol. 48, 1960, pp. 226-253.

[8] Peryam, D. R. and Pilgrim, F. J., *Food Technology,* Vol. 11, 1957, pp. 9-14.

[9] Rubacky, E. P., *The Science of Hedonics–A Work Book,* Waldron Enterprises, Haddonfield, N. J., 1970.

[10] Baker, G. A., Amerine, M. A., and Pangborn, R. M., *Journal of Food Science,* Vol. 26, 1961, pp. 644-647.

[11] Pangborn, R. M. in *The Chemical Senses and Nutrition,* R. Kare and O. Mabler, Eds., The Johns Hopkins Press, Baltimore, 1967, Chapter 4.

[12] *Basic Principles of Sensory Evaluation, ASTM STP 433,* American Society for Testing and Materials, 1968, pp. 7-10.

[13] Cavonius, C. R. and Rubacky, E. P., *Behavior Research Methods and Instrumentation,* Vol. 3, No. 1, 1971, pp. 46-47.

[14] Johnston, J. W., Jr. and Rubacky, E. P., "Futility of Hedonic Appraisals Without an Established Convention," Psychonomic Society, San Antonio, Tex., 5 Nov. 1970, (abstract).

[15] Litchfield, J. T. and Wilcoxon, F. W., *Journal of Pharmacology and Experimental Therapeutics,* Vol. 96, 1949, p. 99.

[16] Conklin, E. S., "The Scale of Values Method for Studies in Genetic Psychology," University of Oregon Publications, Vol. 2, No. 1, 1923.

[17] Johnston, J. W., Jr. and Rubacky, E. P., "Stability of Hedonic Behavior," Psychonomic Society, St. Louis, Mo., 11 Nov. 1971, (abstract).

[18] Johnston, J. W., Jr. and Rubacky, E. P., "Olfactory Hedonics," Society of Cosmetic Chemists, Los Angeles, Calif., 25 May 1972, in press.

[19] Rubacky, E. P., "Report of the Official Survey of Opinions, 1st U. S. International Transportation Exposition (Transpo '72)," Department of Transportation, Federal Aviation Agency, 20 July 1972.

R. M. Pickett [1]

Sensory Evaluation: Potentials for Precision and More General Application in Science and Technology*

REFERENCE: Pickett, R. M., "**Sensory Evaluation: Potentials for Precision and More General Application in Science and Technology,**" *Sensory Evaluation of the Appearance of Materials, ASTM STP 545,* American Society for Testing and Materials, 1973, pp. 185-194.

ABSTRACT: This paper presents a case for devoting increased attention to the refinement and general application of sensory evaluation in science and technology. Today, probably because of immense recent achievements in instrumentation and automation, the scientific and technical community generally looks toward instrumentation to provide measures of objects and events. This inclination may be generally appropriate, but we caution: (1) that it may inhibit seeking significant achievable refinements in current sensory evaluation methods that may have to fill long gaps between now and the time effective instruments are developed; and (2) that it may lead to acceptance of instruments with effectiveness that falls far short of what could be attained with refined sensory evaluation techniques.

KEY WORDS: senses, perception, technological intelligence, astronomy, medicine

Many phenomena now subject to scientific investigation or monitored for technical control might never have been discovered were it not for their initial detection in the experiences of alert and curious human observers. Often, human experience has continued to contribute beyond the point of discovering phenomena to provide scientific and technical data about them in the form of sensory evaluations. Sooner or later, however, the questions that are asked, or

*This paper was written under support from the Public Health Service (Grant #5R01-GM18253-02) and the Air Force (Contract #F19628-71-C-0098).

[1] Formerly, assistant professor of Experimental Psychophysiology, Guggenheim Center for Aerospace Health and Safety, School of Public Health, Harvard University, Boston, Mass. 02115. Now senior scientist, Bolt, Beranek, and Newman, Inc., Cambridge, Mass. 02138.

the controls that are required, become too fine to be answered through crude sensory evaluation, even by the most diligent and acute observers, and progress awaits refinement of the evaluation process. By a refined evaluation process, we mean one that is more narrowly focused on the specific quality of interest, and one that is subject to less drift and noise. The potential for refinement by reducing the effects of noise, or equivalently increasing the precision of evaluation, is the main point of interest here. Here, precision refers to the size of deviations from the mean obtained by repeated application of the evaluation procedure.

The scientific and technical community is strongly inclined to seek refinement through instrumentation. But, while searches in that direction have been enormously rewarding, particularly in recent decades, there are examples in which instrumentation has been very slowly achieved. In the interim, work on improved sensory methods might have permitted substantial progress had it been undertaken. A good modern example of this situation is in the area of medical imagery screening. Decades of work on an automated approach to Pap smear screening have yet to yield an accurate and economical instrument for field operations. Over those same decades there has been no formal effort to refine current sensory evaluation techniques. Yet, a study described in this paper suggests that there is considerable potential for such refinement. Before presenting the Pap smear case, however, a simpler illustration from the field of astronomy will be presented.

A Case Study from Astronomy: Evaluating the Brightness of Stars

Evaluating star brightness as a scientific problem can be traced back to the time of Hipparchus (circa 150 B.C.). From that time until the development of fine optical comparators and of photographic and photometric techniques in the 19th century, star brightness was determined by crude absolute and comparative sensory evaluations. For centuries, sensory evaluation in the form of absolute judgments of magnitude was sufficient for the primary task of constructing star atlases. Individual observers assigned each star to one of six categories of brightness. Apparently from very early on, it was recognized that six categories gave the most precise degree of distinction. It is interesting to find that studies in recent times [*1*] [2] have tended to confirm that situation. Precise distinctions by individual observers are, in fact, limited to about five or six categories when the test stimuli are well spaced on the brightness dimension. Beyond that degree of distinction, the mean square error is such that evaluations for neighboring categories begin to significantly overlap.

By the 17th and 18th centuries, more refined questions about stellar brightness were being asked, first in connection with the problem of establishing

[2] The italic numbers in brackets refer to the list of references appended to this paper.

star distance as a function of brightness, and later in detecting and mapping the periods of variable stars. One approach to refinement was to employ selected stars as standards against which other stars could be compared in brightness. Polaris was frequently used as a standard. Unfortunately, refined methods available only toward the end of the 19th century showed that Polaris itself was a variable star. Another 18th century approach particularly valuable in detecting variable stars was Hershel's method of sequences ([*2*] pp. 347-348). If a group of stars are observed and their order of brightness noted at two different times, then any alteration in the order would show that the brightness of one had changed. Thus, some refinement was achieved beyond the classic six category absolute judgment method, but sensory evaluation was still very crude.

With the development of fine optical comparators early in the 19th century, sensory evaluations were greatly refined. But even here, lack of precision still would have precluded answers to some questions of great interest, for example, about the periods of variable stars. Further refinement of sensory evaluation was sought and achieved through the method of average error. The observer was required to make repeated matches between the brightness of a standard point of light in the comparator and the test star. The average was then made as precise as necessary by increasing the number of individual readings. That method sufficed to produce evaluations of brightness more precise than those that could be obtained by the best photometric techniques until very recently. From that point on, no further improvements in sensory evaluation were required for stellar brightness estimation.

The problem of further refinement in sensory evaluation then fell largely into the hands of sensory physiologists and experimental psychologists, who borrowed the general sensory evaluation approach to study the sensory process itself[*3*], with an aim diametrically opposite to that of the astronomers. The physiologists and psychologists sought measures of sensory structure and function through tests of the detection and discriminability of known stimulus variables. From the earliest studies of sensory structure and function in the middle of the 19th century to the present, sensory evaluation has been greatly refined. It has also been expanded under the general rubric of psychometric methods[*4*], to permit studies of a broad spectrum of human perceptual and judgmental processes as well. Much of this methodology can now, however, be turned back to the task of evaluating unknown qualities of objects and events for general scientific and technical purposes.

The significance of this point can be appreciated in historical perspective by turning again to the problem of stellar brightness estimation. Stevens and Galanter[*5*] applied a highly refined sensory evaluation technique to estimate stellar brightness. They used the method of magnitude estimation, pooling single reports from 15 observers. The task for each observer was to assign numbers proportional to the apparent brightness of the star. The observer could use any number he thought appropriate. The medians of those 15 estimates for each level of star brightness are plotted against luminance in Fig. 1. The figure shows that with this method very precise distinctions can be made in stellar brightness without an optical comparator. This method, which requires no gadgetry at all, could have been used centuries before fine optical comparators were available to detect and map the periods of variable stars.

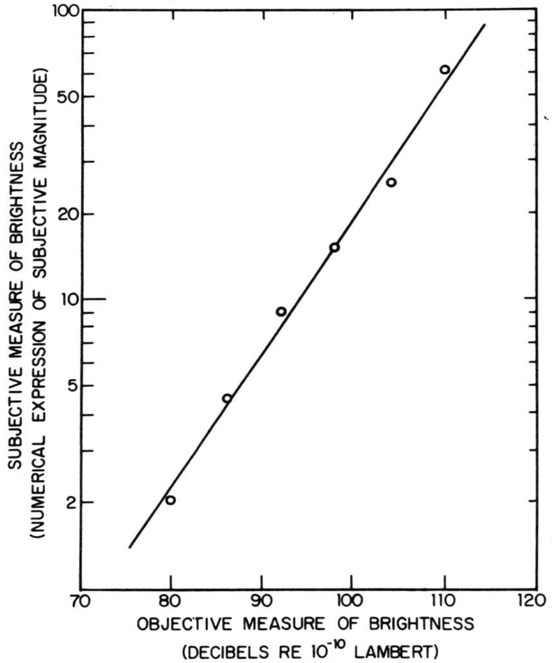

FIG. 1–*Evidence of the potential for precise sensory evaluation of stellar brightness. Each point is the median of 15 independent magnitude estimates. Figure redrawn from Stevens and Galanter*[5].

Magnitude estimation as illustrated in the Stevens and Galanter study is one of many recently developed procedures that can be followed in sensory and perceptual evaluation. A simple and generally applicable method, it permits scaling any quality where one can establish for the observer a sense of a qualitative or quantitative continuum with at least one well placed anchor point. Another general technique called category scaling could also have wide application as is illustrated in the following section.

An Illustration from Medicine: Scaling the Appearance of Pap Smears

To check a Pap smear[6] for evidence of uterine cancer, a lone highly trained observer examines it under a microscope. A smear contains a large number of exfoliated cells, and the observer has to examine them all, looking for ones that are malignant. It is a demanding job, and much effort has gone into research on ways to automate it, largely to no avail.

From examination of many smears, subtle differences in overall appearance between positive and negative smears become apparent, even to naive observers. Professional observers agree that positive and negative smears often do differ in overall appearance, citing cytological and histological factors which account for differences. They insist, however, that such visible differences are too diffuse and subtle, and that their evaluations would not be precise enough for definitive diagnoses. But, clearly, if their evaluations of overall appearance could be made precise, a new and perhaps less onerous method for screening smears might be forthcoming.

In recent studies, employing the method of category scaling (see Ref *5*), naive observers scaled the appearance of Pap smears along four dimensions of overall appearance: opacity, extrudability, explosiveness, and looseness. The format for each of those scales is shown in Fig. 2. For a detailed description of the observer instructions that define each scale, see Ref *7*.

General Procedure

Detailed reports of these studies are in preparation. We present here a general description of the procedure sufficient to show some results of these studies of immediate relation to this article.

Stimuli—The test stimuli came from 75 cervical smears obtained from a local teaching hospital; 25 negative, 25 dysplastic (near malignant) and 25 malignant (carcinoma *in situ*) smears. The positive diagnoses were based on cytological and histopathological analyses by trained medical observers.

Eight 35-mm color photomicrographs (views) were made from each smear. They were taken at a magnification of ×80. Each view constituted about one twenty-fifth the area of a normal microscope field. Each view was chosen by a

FORMAT FOR RATING THE GENERAL APPEARANCE OF PAP SMEARS

1	Transparent	0 1 2 3 4 5 6 7 8 9	Opaque	1
2	Pliable	0 1 2 3 4 5 6 7 8 9	Extrudable	2
		Saran® Wrap (at 1) — Molding Clay (at 8)		
3	Calm	0 1 2 3 4 5 6 7 8 9	Explosive	3
4	Sticky	0 1 2 3 4 5 6 7 8 9	Loose	4
		Saran® Wrap (at 1) — Cellophane (at 8)		

FIG. 2—*Format for category scaling of the overall appearance of Pap smears.*

naive observer, who was instructed to ensure simply that it contained "some material."

Observers—The observers were nine students from Simmons College, who certified that they had had no training of immediate relevance to cytological analysis of Pap smears.

Method—The 35 mm slides were put in one long scrambled sequence in which any one of the eight views of any one of the smears was separated by one view of each of the other 74 smears. The slides were front projected to the students, who were run as a group, but worked independently. The slides were displayed just long enough (5 to 6 s) for all nine observers to rate the displayed section of smear along two dimensions. Over a four-day period each view was shown twice to permit it to be scaled on all four dimensions. One view from each of the 75 smears was scaled twice on each of the dimensions to provide data on precision. The observers recorded their scale values on mark-sense answer sheets.

Data analyses—Data for the precision analysis for each dimension were averages of the scale values given by the nine observers for each view for the first scaling occasion and for the second occasion. The 75 average scale values for each occasion were paired and a Pearson product-moment correlation coefficient was calculated for each dimension as an overall measure of precision.

Data for validity analyses were grand mean scale values for each smear over all views and all observers. Those data were subjected to an analysis-of-variance test.

Results

Precision—Average ratings for the first occasion plotted against average ratings for the second occasion are shown in Fig. 3. The data points cluster closely around the diagonal where they would fall if these data showed no deviation at all on repeated tests.

The correlation coefficients express, in numerical form, this evidence of very high precision. These results are quite remarkable considering the brevity and generality of the observer instructions, the diffuseness of the Pap smear qualities to be assessed, and the immense complexity of the stimuli.

The fact that averaging over nine observers can produce reliable scalings of such general and diffuse qualities is the main point for this discussion. Whether the particular dimensions that were scaled are valid is another interesting, but subsidiary question. After all, the human observer can see many qualities in complex displays like Pap smears, and if the observers had not been aimed at valid dimensions of analysis this time, it is quite probable that with continued explorations some valid dimensions would be found. As it turns out, however, the dimensions did show some validity.

Validity—By validity we mean that the perceived differences have some potential theoretical or practical significance. In this case the basic question is whether the malignant, dysplastic, and negative smears tended to fall at different locations on one or another of the scaled dimensions.

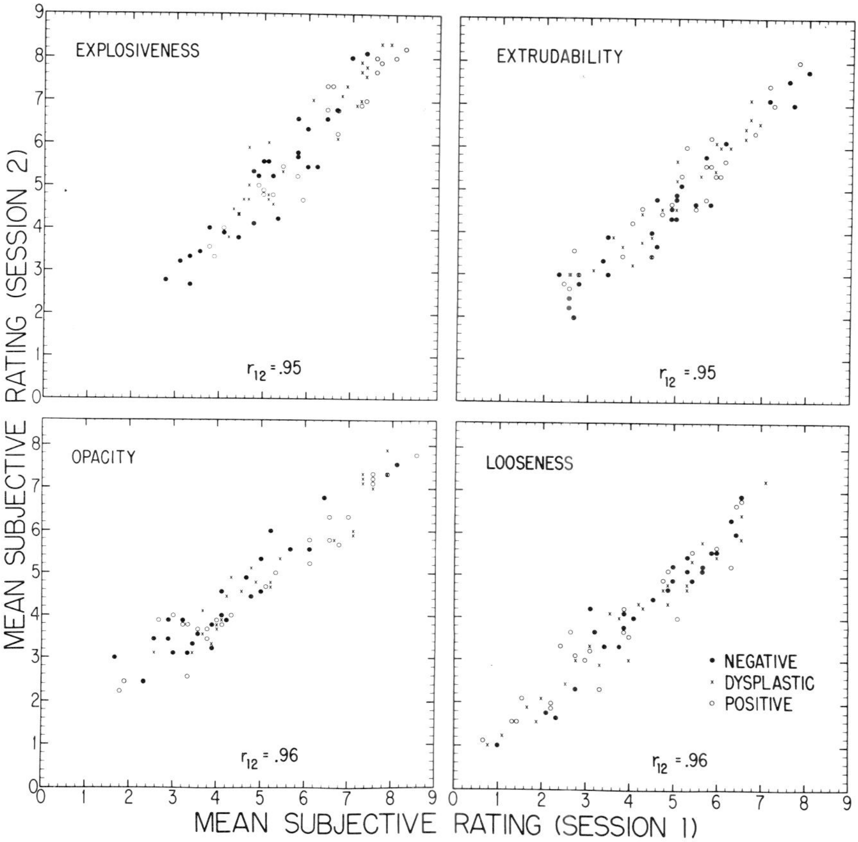

FIG. 3—*Evidence of the potential for precise sensory evaluation of the overall appearance of Pap smears. Each point is the mean of nine independent ratings.*

An analysis of variance, done on the data from each dimension separately, shows that the diagnostic classes are statistically distinguishable on three of the dimensions: explosiveness, opacity, and looseness. A picture of their general positioning on the subjective scales is given in Fig. 4. Shown are the grand mean scale values over all smears in each diagnostic class.

The degree of statistical separation found on each of these dimensions is not sufficient to be of practical significance, although as statistical sampling theory would suggest [*8*], by increasing the number of observations it might be made so. It all depends on how much of the error is due to noise in the sensory evaluation process and how much is due to noise in the smear data. Also, even if error could be reduced to a point of practical significance by increasing the number of sensory evaluations, it might require so many that it would not be practical. A

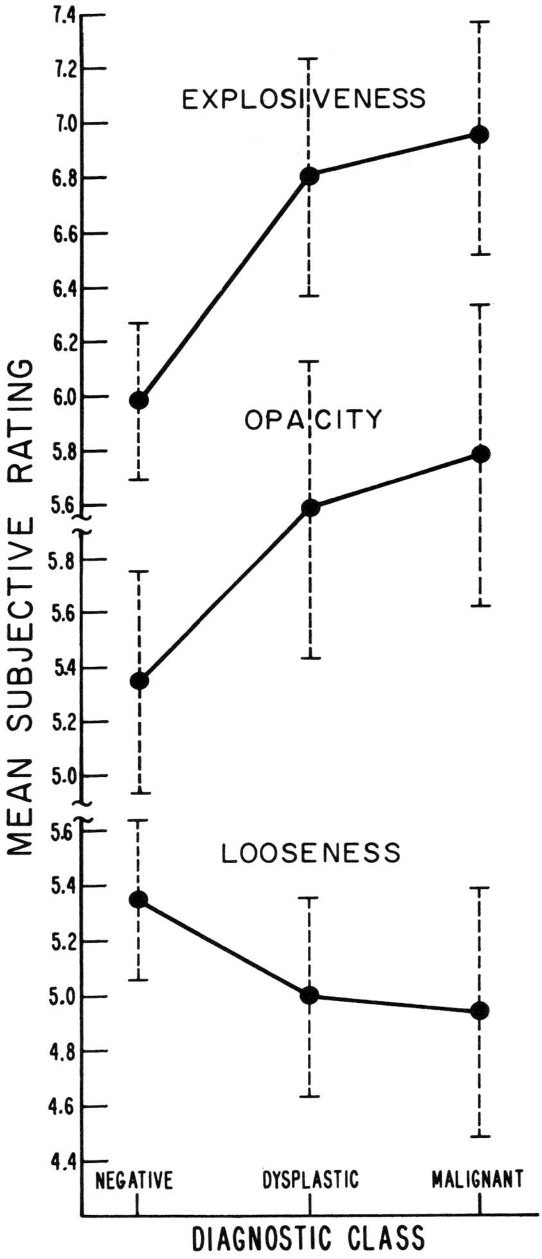

FIG. 4–*Evidence of validity of sensory evaluation of the overall appearance of Pap smears. Shown is the grand mean rating for each diagnostic category. Each point is based on 1800 independent ratings. The length of the dashed lines indicate the range of variability (two standard deviations) for individual smears.*

modest amount of further study could answer that question. These immediate findings, however, may be of theoretical significance, because they demonstrate that there are general and diffuse properties of smears that change as cancer develops.

Summary

Development and use of psychometric methods to enhance sensory evaluation took place before psychology was born; yet, most of the subsequent development and application of these methods has been made in psychology. Psychometric methods, particularly ones developed over the last several decades, could be of great general use to provide precise evaluations of objects and events in many areas of science and technology.

The human observer can sense and assess a very broad range of qualities, including many that are very subtle, diffuse, and complex. Methods like magnitude estimation permit very general use of that human capacity. Statistical sampling theory suggests, and the previous examples show, that large gains in accuracy can come from pooling repeated independent evaluations.

Of great practical significance is the fact that sensory and perceptual evaluations obtained by these techniques need not be limited to simple properties like brightness, color, or size, where human assessment is often superfluous because physical measurement techniques are available. Methods like magnitude estimation and category scaling can be applied to evaluate a very wide range of properties; almost any property in which the human observer can sense systematic variations.

The spectrum of problem areas in science and technology that might benefit from the application of refined sensory evaluation techniques is extremely broad. For example, there are medical applications, such as the auditory assessment of lung and vascular systems. There are scientific applications as in the visual assessment of solar imagery [*9*]. There are also numerous commercial applications, not only in food and flavor evaluation, which is well developed, but also in raw material and general product evaluation.

Human observers are usually interested in contributing their perceptual talents and often derive intrinsic satisfaction from such work. The challenge is to take advantage of their talents in scientific and technical settings where they can be of great use in the absence of other appropriate instruments.

References

[*1*] Ericksen, C. W. and Hake, H. W., *Journal of Experimental Psychology,* Vol. 49, 1955, pp. 323-332.
[*2*] Berry, A., *A Short History of Astronomy,* 1898, Dover, New York, 1961.
[*3*] Titchener, E. B., *Experimental Psychology,* Vol. II, Parts I and II, Macmillan, New York, 1905.
[*4*] Guilford, J. P., *Psychometric Methods,* 2nd ed, McGraw-Hill, New York, 1954.

[5] Stevens, S. S. and Galanter, E. H., *Journal of Experimental Psychology,* Vol. 54, 1957, pp. 377-411.
[6] Papanicolaou, G. N., *Atlas of Exfoliative Cytology,* Harvard University Press, Cambridge, Mass., 1954.
[7] Pickett, R. M., "Applications of Texture Perception in the Analysis of Complex Optical Imagery," Aerospace Medical Research Laboratories Technical Report, AMRL-TR-71-81, May 1972.
[8] Cochran, W. G., *Sampling Techniques,* Wiley, New York, 1953.
[9] Pickett, R. M., "On Enhancing Visual Perceptions of Solar Flare Precursors," Air Force Cambridge Research Laboratories Technical Report, AFCRL-TR-73-0210, April 1973.